The Effective Management of Lung Cancer

Edited by

Martin F Muers MA DPhil FRCP
Consultant Physician, Respiratory Unit, The General Infirmary at Leeds, Leeds, UK

Fergus Macbeth MA DM FRCR FRCP
Director, Clinical Effectiveness Support Unit (Wales), Llandough Hospital, Penarth, Vale of Glamorgan, UK

Francis C Wells MA(Cantab) MS(Lond) MB BS(Hons) FRCS(Eng)
Consultant Cardiothoracic Surgeon, Papworth Hospital, Cambridge, UK

Andrew Miles MSc MPhil PhD
*Professor of Public Health Policy and Health Services Research
& UK Key Advances Series Organiser,
University of East London, UK*

UeL University Centre for Public Health Policy & Health Services Research	Royal College of Radiologists	British Thoracic Society	The Association of Cancer Physicians	Society of Cardiothoracic Surgeons

AESCULAPIUS MEDICAL PRESS
LONDON SAN FRANCISCO SYDNEY

Published by

Aesculapius Medical Press (London, San Francisco, Sydney)
Centre for Public Health Policy and Health Services Research
Faculty of Science and Health
University of East London
33 Shore Road, London E9 7TA, UK

© Aesculapius Medical Press 2001

First published 2001

British Library Cataloguing in Publication Data
A catalogue record for this book is available from the British Library

ISBN 1 903044 12 X

While the advice and information in this book are believed to be true and accurate at the
time of going to press, neither the authors nor the publishers nor the sponsoring institutions
can accept any legal responsibility or liability for any errors or omissions that may be made.
In particular (but without limiting the generality of the preceding disclaimer) every effort
has been made to check drug usages; however, it is possible that errors have been missed.
Furthermore, dosage schedules are constantly being revised and new side-effects recognised.
For these reasons, the reader is strongly urged to consult the drug companies' printed
instructions before administering any of the drugs recommended in this book.

Further copies of this volume are available from:

Claudio Melchiorri
Research Dissemination Fellow
Centre for Public Health Policy and Health Services Research
Faculty of Science and Health
University of East London
33 Shore Road, London E9 7TA, UK

Fax: 020 8525 8661
email: claudio@keyadvances4.demon.co.uk

Typeset, printed and bound in Britain
Peter Powell Origination & Print Limited

The Effective Management of Lung Cancer

Contents

Contributors

Rhada Bhaskaran MRCP, Specialist Registrar in Medical Oncology, CRC Department of Medical Oncology, Christie Hospital and Holt Radium Institute, Manchester, UK

Jessica Corner PhD BSc RGN, Director and Deputy Dean (Nursing), Centre for Cancer and Palliative Care Studies, Institute of Cancer Research, Royal Marsden Hospital, London, UK

Graham G Dark PhD MRCP, Senior Lecturer in Medical Oncology and Cancer Education, University of Newcastle and Northern Centre for Cancer Treatment, Newcastle-upon-Tyne

John G Edwards FRCS(Glasg.), Specialist Registrar in Cardiothoracic Surgery, Department of Thoracic Surgery, Glenfield Hospital, Leicester, UK

Tim Eisen PhD MRCP, Senior Lecturer in Medical Oncology, Department of Oncology, Royal Free and University College Medical School, London, UK

Stephen Falk MB ChB MRCP FRCR MD, Consultant Clinical Oncologist, Bristol Oncology Centre, Bristol, UK

David Forman BA PhD MFPHM, Professor of Cancer Epidemiology, University of Leeds and Director of Research and Information, Northern and Yorkshire Cancer Registry and Information Service, Leeds, UK

Anna Gregor FRCP FRCR, Macmillan Lead Cancer Clinician, Western General Hospital, Edinburgh, UK

Robert A Haward MB ChB DPH FFPHM QHP, Professor of Cancer Studies, University of Leeds and Medical Director, Northern and Yorkshire Cancer Registry and Information Service, Leeds, UK

Sacha J Howell MRCP, Specialist Registrar in Medical Oncology, CRC Department of Medical Oncology, Christie Hospital and Holt Radium Institute, Manchester, UK

Clare Laroche MBBS BSc MD FRCP, Consultant, Respiratory Medicine, Thoracic Oncology Unit, Papworth and Addenbrooke's NHS Trusts, Cambridge, UK

Erica Lowry BA(Hons) RGN RCNT, Macmillan Thoracic Nurse Specialist, Papwoth Hospital, Cambridge, UK

Fergus Macbeth MA DM FRCR FRCP, Director, Clinical Effectiveness Support Unit (Wales), Llandough Hospital, Penarth, Vale of Glamorgan, UK

Mark R Middleton MRCP PhD, CRC Senior Clinical Research Fellow, CRC Department of Medical Oncology, Christie Hospital and Holt Radium Institute, Manchester, UK

Martin F Muers MA DPhil FRCP, Consultant Physician, Respiratory Unit, The General Infirmary at Leeds, Leeds, UK

Marianne C Nicholson MD BSc FRCP(Ed), Consultant Medical Oncologist, ANCHOR Unit, Aberdeen Royal Infirmary, Aberdeen, UK

Mary O'Brien MD FRCP, Consultant Medical Oncologist, Kent Cancer Centre, Maidstone and Royal Marsden NHS Trust, Sutton, UK

Roderick JH Robertson MB ChB MRCP FRCR, Consultant Radiologist, Department of Clinical Radiology, The General Infirmary at Leeds, Leeds, UK

Robin M Rudd MD FRCP, Consultant in Medical Oncology, Department of Medical Oncology, St Bartholomew's Hospital, London, UK

Peter Simmonds MB BS FRACP, Senior Lecturer in Medical Oncology, CRC Wessex Medical Oncology Unit, Southampton General Hospital, Southampton, UK

Jeremy PC Steele MD MRCP, Specialist Registrar, Department of Medical Oncology, St Bartholomew's Hospital, London, UK

Nicholas Thatcher PhD FRCP, Professor of Medical Oncology, CRC Department of Medical Oncology, Christie Hospital and Holt Radium Institute, Manchester, UK

David A Waller FRCS(CTh), Consultant Thoracic Surgeon, Department of Thoracic Surgery, Glenfield Hospital, Leicester, UK

Francis C Wells MA(Cantab) MS(Lond) MB BS(Hons) FRCS(Eng), Consultant Cardiothoracic Surgeon, Papworth Hospital, Cambridge, UK

Preface

Lung cancer, causing nearly 40,000 deaths annually in the UK and affecting more women now than breast cancer, remains the most frequent of all malignant diseases and the one with the poorest prognosis. However, after many years of nihilism and static survival figures, recent data, summarised in this volume, has shown a welcome improvement both in life expectancy and in the quality of life of treated patients.

These advances have, in part, been due to organisational shifts following the Calman-Hine proposals, and to a better appreciation of the fact that all patients can benefit from the application of the major therapeutic modalities – lung cancer surgery, radiotherapy and chemotherapy, together with combined modality treatment.

It is important for state-of-the-art, contemporary summaries, such as this volume, to look forward and to anticipate developments. The attention of readers, in this respect, is particularly directed to the chapter on screening by Eisen. Since so many patients with lung cancer, most of whom are over 70 years old, present with advanced disease, there is no realistic prospect of a quantum improvement in prognosis unless the disease can be routinely detected earlier in its trajectory. Although trials of screening by chest x-ray and sputum cytology in the 1970s and 1980s have long been regarded as negative, the advent of low-cost spiral CT for peripheral lesions and cytogenetic tests for cellular abnormalities in sputum and blood are about to change this perspective fundamentally. A later edition of this volume is certain to contain much new information from the results of the new screening trials currently being set up around the world.

Two other areas of rapid change also claim particular mention. The first is chemotherapy for inoperable disease. This treatment is developing a large evidence base and is likely to become a standard approach for many patients in the near future. Corner's chapter also shows how, amidst pharmaceutical and organisational change, the holistic approach to patients' symptoms by specialist nurses can produce grades of improvement in quality of life which are large and devoid of toxicity.

In the current age, where doctors and health professionals are increasingly overwhelmed by clinical information, we have aimed to provide a fully current, fully referenced text which is as succinct as possible, but as comprehensive as necessary. Consultants in surgical, medical and clinical oncology, and in respiratory and thoracic medicine, and their trainees, will find it of particular use as part of their continuing professional development and specialist training, and we advance it explicitly as an excellent tool for these purposes. We anticipate, however, that the book will also prove of use to clinical nurse specialists as a reference text and to commissioners of health services as the basis for discussion and negotiation of health contracts with their practising colleagues.

In conclusion, we thank Eli-Lilly & Co. Ltd for the grant of educational sponsorship which helped organise a national symposium held with the Royal College of

Radiologists, the British Thoracic Society, The Association of Cancer Physicians and the Society of Cardiothoracic Surgeons at the Royal College of Physicians of London, at which synopses of the constituent chapters of this book were presented.

Martin F Muers MA DPhil FRCP
Fergus Macbeth MA DM FRCR FRCP
Francis C Wells MA(Cantab) MS(Lond) MB BS(Hons) FRCS(Eng)
Andrew Miles MSc MPhil PhD

PART 1

Epidemiology, screening and quality of care

Chapter 1

The health care epidemiology of lung cancer

Robert A Haward and David Forman

Introduction

The publication by the Department of Health in 1995 of *A Policy Framework for Commissioning Cancer Services* marked a watershed in English cancer policy. For the first time there was a clear policy framework for the delivery of cancer services. This covered all sites of cancer and all parts of the health care system, encompassing primary care, local hospitals and tertiary centres. One of the main themes of this policy was the need to ensure all patients had access to specialists in the disease in question, and that specialists with interests in particular cancers should work effectively together in multidisciplinary clinical teams. It must be appreciated that this policy marked a radical departure from previous practice in most of the country. The objective of improving clinical organisation and practice was based on a review of evidence about the way that care had previously been organised (Selby *et al.* 1996).

For lung cancer, the subsequent national guidance *Improving Outcomes in Lung Cancer* (Department of Health 1998) made it clear that the necessary specialist teams would be in cancer units and in cancer centres (in respect of their local service), with access to tertiary services required for thoracic surgery and radiotherapy. The guidance identified the key changes required to implement modern multidisciplinary team working. It enabled local services to be appraised against requirements set out in the guidance and allowed local priorities for service development to be accurately determined.

Population-based evidence about patterns of cancer care, and their relationship to outcomes, provides an important means of assessing past services and over time will enable the monitoring of changes in the processes and outcomes of new patterns of service delivery. Studies based on the analysis of data from cancer registries, are potentially more reliable than institutional studies in revealing such patterns of service delivery, precisely as a result of their population-based focus. They are, therefore, less likely to omit patients whose care is atypical, based outside the hospital system, or who die before care is initiated. The main weaknesses are that information about clinical case-mix and the nature or place of treatment is often limited. Not all registries, for example, record relevant information on access to specialised care and specific treatment modalities. In lung cancer in particular, the poor prognosis for most patients, with the resulting short survival after presentation, makes rapid access to care critical to any attempt to improve outcomes.

The former Yorkshire Cancer Registry – now part of the Northern and Yorkshire Cancer Registry and Information Service (NYCRIS), has a substantial, high quality dataset about lung cancer collected over more than 20 years. The former Yorkshire health region (population 3.6 million) is large and diverse enough to reveal variations in services and outcomes. The registry routinely records information about patient contacts with the Health Service, the extent to which diagnosis is confirmed histologically, and the principal modalities of treatment those patients receive. This enables population based analysis of these issues with large numbers of patients over a considerable time period. This type of data has recently been published for lung cancer as part of a series of reports arising from an NHS research and development funded registry based research project for the Yorkshire region (the key sites study) (Cancer Outcomes Monitoring 1999). This study used large numbers of lung cancer patients (22,600 patients over eight years from 1986 to 1994). In addition, an active group of regional clinicians with interests in lung cancer have worked with the cancer registry on a study of lung cancer referral patterns, which is also available in report form (Cancer Outcomes Monitoring 2000). Taken together, data from the registry study of lung cancer and the lung referral study allow a population-based analysis of the main features of access and care. The data are summarised in this chapter. The full reports containing these data are published by NYCRIS, and copies can be obtained on request or downloaded from the website.[1] Appropriate scientific papers for peer-reviewed journals are being submitted.

Access to care

The principal source of information about access to lung cancer services is derived from a study based on a random sample of 400 lung cancer patients drawn from across the region (Cancer Outcomes Monitoring 2000). In order to ensure a representative sample the patients were stratified by age, sex and district health authority of residence. In addition to this study the large cohort of all lung cancer registrations prepared for the key sites study was analysed for some of the same characteristics, and was therefore available to be compared with the referral sample. Thus, data from the complete population enabled validation of the sample. It was shown to mirror the wider population very closely.

Table 1.1 shows the patient characteristics of lung cancer referrals in the sample by sex, age group and tumour type. The cases were divided into three clinical presentation categories based on review of both primary care and hospital case-notes. The first, headed 'with diagnosis' comprised patients whose symptoms led the GP to order a chest x-ray which showed a radiological diagnosis suggesting lung cancer, enabling the GP referral to be made with a presumptive diagnosis of lung cancer.

---

[1]   Copies of the two reports referred to in this chapter are available free of charge.
    They can be downloaded from the cancer registry web-site: http://www.nycris.org.uk
    They can also be obtained by writing to the Information Manager, NYCRIS, Arthington House,
    Hospital Lane, Leeds LS16 6QB.

The second group, 'without diagnosis' were patients with very varied symptomatology, including, but not necessarily dominated by, respiratory symptoms, in whom no chest x-ray was performed in primary care, and in which the referral from the GP was not based on a diagnosis of lung cancer. The third group, headed 'acute' were patients who were not referred by their GP in the conventional way, but who presented to Accident and Emergency, or were otherwise admitted as emergencies.

Table 1.1 also shows the frequency of the two main histological categories in the sample, small cell and non-small cell, together with a third category labelled 'clinical'. This latter group were those for whom there was no histological or cytological confirmation of lung cancer, but in whom management was based on a clinical diagnosis of lung cancer. The number of patients studied – 362 – represented those in the sample for whom both primary care and hospital records were available for analysis. There were a few cases in which one or other set of records could not be traced and these were omitted from the study, as were death certificate only registrations of lung cancer.

The most important conclusion from Table 1.1 is the fact that slightly less than half lung cancer patients presented with what might be regarded as a typical lung cancer presentation. Many guidelines (Standing Medical Advisory Committee 1994; British Thoracic Society 1998; Scottish Intercollegiate Guidelines Network 1998;

Table 1.1 Summary of patient characteristics in the referrals sample study and within three presentation groups [1993 incident sample]

Factor		All cases		With diagnosis		Without diagnosis		Acute	
		n	%	n	%	n	%	n	%
Sex	Male	226	62.4	105	60.7	97	65.5	24	58.5
	Female	136	37.6	68	39.3	51	34.5	17	41.5
Age group	<65	96	26.5	44	25.4	41	27.7	11	26.8
	65–75	153	42.3	85	49.1	49	33.1	19	46.3
	75+	113	31.2	44	25.4	58	39.2	11	26.8
Histological confirmation	Yes	247	68.2	139	80.3	87	58.8	21	48.8
	No	115	31.8	34	19.7	61	41.2	20	51.2
Tumour type	Non-Small Cell	185	51.1	112	64.7	60	40.5	13	31.7
	Small Cell	62	17.1	27	15.6	27	18.2	8	19.5
	Clinical	115	31.8	34	19.7	61	41.2	20	48.8
Total cases in each group	% in each group of all cases	362	100.0	173	47.8	148	40.9	41	11.3

Department of Health 2000) focus particularly on the patient with respiratory symptoms presenting in primary care, on whom a chest x-ray is performed, as if that is the only pathway for lung cancer patients to be referred to hospital. This study demonstrates that although this is the largest single group, it accounts for less than half the total lung cancer workload in hospitals. Elderly patients in this study were more likely to be in the group without diagnosis, a finding discussed more fully later.

Table 1.2 shows the specialty of the consultant to whom the GP initially referred the patient, or, in the case of acute admissions, the speciality of the consultant who had initial responsibility for that patient's management. This demonstrates that the typical 'with diagnosis' group of patients was predominantly (87 per cent) referred directly to respiratory disease specialists, either to chest physicians or, in a few cases, to thoracic surgeons. Both specialities can be regarded as appropriate for the management of lung cancer. The remaining 13 per cent of these patients were referred to other specialists, normally physicians, without a specialist role in lung cancer.

The 'without diagnosis' group, as might be anticipated, showed an extremely varied pattern of initial referral. The largest single specialty group, accounting for about a third of these patients, was physicians in medicine for the elderly. Less than a quarter of these patients were initially referred to an appropriate speciality for lung cancer management. The acute patients revealed a particularly wide range of managing specialities at the hospital, including a range of surgical specialties, no doubt reflecting the variety of clinical presentations.

However, whilst the pattern of these initial referrals illustrates the chosen route of GPs, and reveals important information about the point of first contact in hospital, it is not the whole story. It is necessary to understand whether or not these patients were subsequently referred on to specialists in lung cancer, once their diagnosis became apparent.

Table 1.2 Speciality of first consultant by presentation group [1993 incident sample]

Speciality	All cases		With diagnosis		Without diagnosis		Acute	
	n	%	n	%	n	%	n	%
Chest physician	180	49.7	141	81.5	33	22.3	6	14.6
Thoracic surgeon	9	2.5	9	5.2	0	0.0	0	0.0
General medicine	54	14.9	12	6.9	30	20.3	12	29.3
Medicine for the elderly	58	16	8	4.6	45	30.4	5	12.2
General surgery	15	4.1	2	1.2	10	6.8	3	7.3
Other	46	12.7	1	0.6	30	20.3	15	36.6
Totals	362	100.0	173	100.0	148	100.0	41	100.0

Table 1.3 Specialist management by presentation group [1993 incident sample]

Specialist management	All cases		With diagnosis		Without diagnosis		Acute	
	n	%	n	%	n	%	n	%
Managed by a specialist	284	78.4	166	96.0	93	62.8	25	61
Opinion given but not managed by a specialist	46	12.7	4	2.3	34	23.0	8	20
No specialist management or opinion	32	8.8	3	1.7	21	14.2	8	20
Total	362	100.0	173	100.0	148	100.0	41	100.0

Table 1.3 summarises the extent to which patients came under the management of a lung cancer specialist or, if not under their direct management, whether a specialist opinion was made available by appropriate specialists in lung cancer to the clinical team responsible for their management. In this context a specialist is a respiratory physician, a thoracic surgeon, or a clinical oncologist.

In the 'with diagnosis' group, a high proportion of whom were first referred to a relevant specialist, almost all (96 per cent) obtained specialist management, with less than 2 per cent receiving neither specialist management nor a specialist opinion. In the 'without diagnosis' group almost two thirds of cases came under specialist management and almost a quarter had a specialist opinion, although not under specialist management. However, one in seven (14.2 per cent) of these patients received neither a specialist opinion, nor came under specialist management at any time. This represents an important subgroup that need to be brought within specialist care as part of the implementation of national cancer policy. This is specifically recommended[3] in the national cancer guidance, *Improving Outcomes in Lung cancer* (Department of Health 1998). The 'acute' group showed a similar pattern to the 'without diagnosis' group, although the proportion receiving neither a specialist opinion, nor coming under specialist management, was higher at one in five of the group.

These differences in the extent to which patients referred in different ways were able to access a lung cancer specialist continued in relationship to diagnostic practice. Table 1.4 shows that the frequency with which patients were bronchoscoped was much lower in the 'without diagnosis' group (60.1 per cent) and the 'acute' group (56.1 per cent) than the 'with diagnosis' group in whom 85 per cent had this procedure. Mediastinoscopy, which is often part of the detailed clinical assessment for possible radical treatment, was carried out in 8.7 per cent of the 'with diagnosis' group, but in only 1.4 per cent of the 'without diagnosis' and 2.4 per cent of the 'acute' group. The frequency of CT scans is similar across the three groups. This suggests that diagnostic modalities requiring the active involvement of lung cancer specialists are

Table 1.4 Diagnostic investigations by presentation group [1993 incident sample]

Investigation	All cases		With diagnosis		Without diagnosis		Acute	
	n	%	n	%	n	%	n	%
Bronchoscopy	236	73.5	147	85.0	89	60.1	23	56.1
Mediastinoscopy	17	5.3	15	8.7	2	1.4	1	2.4
CT Scan	130	40.5	75	43.4	55	37.2	17	41.0

less likely to be performed in the patient groups that are less often referred initially to lung cancer specialists. CT, a more generic form of hospital diagnostic investigation, is equally likely whatever the speciality of initial referral.

The large registry-based population study of lung cancer from 1986–1994 demonstrated almost identical rates of overall specialist management (74.5 per cent, compared to 78.4 per cent in the referral study). Table 1.5, taken from the population study, demonstrates that histological confirmation in the specialist-managed group of patients was 77.4 per cent, but only 33.7 per cent in those not receiving any specialist management. The registry data did not show whether or not patients who didn't receive specialist management might have had access to a specialist opinion. Histological confirmation of the cell type in lung cancer is nearly always necessary for the determination of the most appropriate management.

Table 1.6 illustrates the histological confirmation rates by sex, age, and socio-economic status for successive three-year time periods. There was a small difference between male and female histological confirmation rates, with confirmation being slightly more likely in males. The age distribution showed a strong trend in relation to age for histological confirmation with a fall in rates between the under-65s and 65–74 age groups, from 81.6 per cent to 70.5 per cent and a much larger drop to 45.9 per cent in patients aged 75 and over.

Table 1.5 Proportion of patients managed by at least one lung cancer specialist: showing histological confirmation rates and disease type: 1986–1994

Specialist/ non-specialist	All		*Histological Confirmation Rate	Confirmed small cell		Confirmed non-small cell		Clinically diagnosed	
	n	%	%	n	%	n	%	n	%
Specialist managed	16884	74.5	77.4	2172	88.7	10899	86.7	3813	49.9
No specialist management	5770	25.5	33.7	276	11.3	1671	13.3	3823	50.1
Total	22654	100	66.3	2448	10.8	12570	55.5	7636	33.7

Table 1.6 Histological confirmation rates by sex, age, socioeconomic status and time: 1986–1994.

Factor		n	Histologically confirmed		Clinically diagnosed	
			n	%	n	%
Overall	N	22,654	15,018	66.3	7,636	33.7
Sex	Male	15,229	10247	67.3	4982	32.7
	Female	7,425	4771	64.3	2654	35.7
Age	<65	6,733	5,491	81.6	1,242	18.4
	65–74	8,995	6,345	70.5	2,650	29.5
	75+	6,926	3,182	45.9	3,744	54.1
Socio-economic status	1–3	3,559	2,379	66.8	1180	33.2
	4–7	12,542	8,238	65.7	4304	34.3
	8–10	6,525	4,382	67.2	2143	32.8
Time period	86–88	7583	4703	62.0	2880	38.0
	89–91	7586	5090	67.1	2496	32.9
	92–94	7485	5225	69.8	2260	30.2

The socioeconomic status classification used is 'Super-Profiles' (Brown & Batey 1994). This is a proprietary system based on the evaluation of 120 census variables at Enumeration District level, many of which are highly correlated. These were analysed by principal components analysis followed by cluster analysis, to derive relatively homogenous profile groups. This process was used to define an initial group of 160 homogenous profile groups which were then refined further down to just ten groups, the 'Super Profiles'.

The classification revealed the expected socioeconomic gradient in incidence (not shown) between the most advantaged super-profile groups (1–3), and the least advantaged (8–10). There was a negligible difference in histological confirmation rates by socio-economic status. This is an important observation, given the pronounced socio-economic variation in incidence of the disease, and in the light of current Health Service policy concerns with equity in access to high quality care. It showed that access to a proper tissue diagnosis was equally likely across the socioeconomic spectrum.

Table 1.6 shows that histological confirmation rates rose in successive time periods in this study from 62 per cent in the period 1986–1988 to almost 70 per cent in the most recent period 1992–1994. There is also substantial variation in these histological confirmation rates by district of residence, as can be seen in Figure 1.1. The rates for both younger and older patients varied by about 18 per cent between the highest and lowest districts, and there was no obvious relationship between rates in older and younger patients in individual districts.

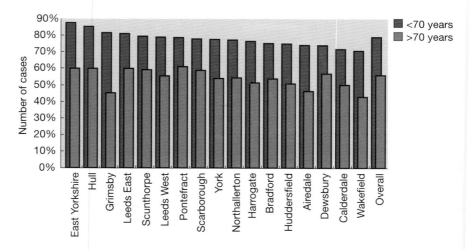

Figure 1.1 Histological confirmation rates by district of residence and age group: 1986–1994.

Current national policy for rapid access for urgent cancer cases (Department of Health 2000) (the two-week wait for urgent referrals) has concentrated attention on the time taken between referral by a GP and the first appointment in the hospital. Yorkshire Cancer Registry data for the period 1994–1996 (not shown) demonstrated a median interval for lung cancer of only ten days. However, the median delay between first hospital appointment and start of treatment showed a median delay in lung cancer of 43 days. In one quarter of all lung cancer patients this interval is longer than 71 days. These hospital delay figures are poorer than for other common cancers, with the exception of prostate cancer, which has a similar median delay but a longer tail to the distribution.

The key conclusions about access to care for lung cancer patients in the UK are therefore that, in 1993:

- just under one half of all lung cancer patients presented to hospital with a suspected diagnosis of lung cancer;
- a significant minority of lung cancer patients did not see a specialist in lung cancer or receive a specialist opinion;
- patients initially referred without a diagnosis or admitted acutely were less likely to see a specialist, to have received a bronchoscopy or mediastinoscopy or to have had their diagnosis histologically confirmed, than were patients initially referred with a radiological diagnosis of lung cancer;
- histological confirmation rates declined substantially with age and also varied slightly by sex; there was variation between different health authority populations;

- whilst access to hospital was reasonably quick once the GP had decided to make a referral, there were substantial delays between patients being first seen and the initiation of their treatment.

Treatment

Table 1.7 shows patterns of treatment for the main subtypes of lung cancer by type of treatment and by age. The column headed 'none' refers to the absence of active treatment of the lung cancer, as distinct from the provision of supportive care. It is not possible from routine cancer registry data to accurately determine the therapeutic intent of treatment, i.e., to distinguish between radical and palliative radiotherapy, chemotherapy or surgery. However, it can be presumed that the data for chemotherapy in small cell lung cancer, and for surgery in non-small cell lung cancer, will reflect treatment with radical intent in a large proportion of cases.

Table 1.7 Treatment practices by age group: 1986–1994

Type	Age	Total	Any S		Any Ch		Any RT		None	
			n	%	n	%	n	%	n	%
Confirmed	<65	1012	34	3.4	693	68.5	451	44.6	186	18.4
small	65–74	1039	24	2.3	563	54.2	389	37.4	309	29.7
cell	75+	397	7	1.8	94	23.7	110	27.7	218	54.9
Confirmed	<65	4479	1216	27.1	393	8.8	2299	51.3	1132	25.3
non-small	65–74	5306	1002	18.9	217	4.1	2379	44.8	2002	37.7
cell	75+	2785	181	6.5	71	2.5	950	34.1	1627	58.4
Clinically	<65	1242	10	0.8	59	4.8	439	35.3	770	62.0
diagnosed	65–74	2650	10	0.4	34	1.3	669	25.2	1950	73.6
	75+	3744	2	0.1	18	0.5	446	11.9	3279	87.6

S= surgery, RT= radiotherapy, Ch = chemotherapy

Treatment rates declined significantly across the age groups with smaller proportions of the over-75s receiving any of these treatment modalities in comparison to the under-65s. Those in whom the diagnosis was not histologically confirmed (i.e., the clinically diagnosed group) had much lower rates of treatment than either of the patient groups with a confirmed histological diagnosis. These figures included radiotherapy, most of which was given with palliative intent.

Figure 1.2 shows treatment rates on a geographical basis by district of residence. The fourth column shows the proportion of lung cancer patients who received any of the principal treatment modalities (surgery, chemotherapy and radiotherapy). The overall active treatment rates varied from just over one third (34.2 per cent) to over a half (56.1 per cent). The treatment rates for any specific modality varied by a

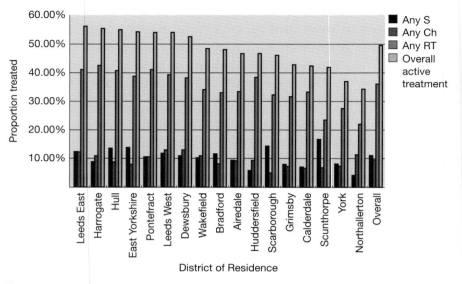

Figure 1.2 District treatment rates (%) 1986–1994.

factor of two for surgery (discounting the very low rate for Northallerton, which is believed to be an under-estimate, based on extra regional referrals). There was a slightly larger proportionate difference for chemotherapy from a low of 5 per cent to a high of 12.9 per cent, and for radiotherapy the range was from 21.9–42.6 per cent. Looking specifically at the main potentially radical treatments, the range for chemotherapy in confirmed small cell lung cancer was from 42.2–81.0 per cent and that for surgery in non-small cell lung cancer varied from 10.5–22.7 per cent. This again showed an approximately two-fold variation in each case. These data are based on districts of residence, not districts of treatment, and reflect quite large differences in the extent to which particular populations received the main treatment modalities in lung cancer.

Table 1.8 shows the treatment modality proportions by socioeconomic group. There was no real difference. Taken together with the data about histological confirmation (Table 1.6), this showed that there is no difference in diagnosis or treatment between socio-economic groups despite the large socio-economic gradient in incidence.

The key conclusions about treatment of lung cancer patients are therefore that, between 1986 and 1994:

- treatment rates declined sharply with age, but did not vary by social class or by sex (data not shown);
- those in whom the type of lung cancer was not histologically diagnosed were less likely to receive active treatment for their lung cancer;

Table 1.8 Treatment practices by socioeconomic group: 1986–1994

Socio-economic group		Total	Any S n	Any S %	Any Ch n	Any Ch %	Any RT n	Any RT %	None n	None %
Confirmed	1–3	361	13	3.6	188	52.1	134	37.1	116	32.1
small	4–7	1315	39	3.0	724	55.1	510	38.8	379	28.8
cell	8–10	770	13	1.7	437	56.8	304	39.5	218	28.3
Confirmed	1–3	2018	385	19.1	126	6.2	879	43.6	792	39.2
non-small	4–7	6923	1337	19.3	376	5.4	3100	44.8	2606	37.6
cell	8–10	3612	673	18.6	178	4.9	1642	45.5	1357	37.6
Clinically	1–3	1180	5	0.4	22	1.9	218	18.5	947	80.3
diagnosed	4–7	4304	13	0.3	71	1.6	905	21.0	3344	77.7
	8–10	2143	4	0.2	18	0.8	429	20.0	1701	79.4

S= surgery, RT= radiotherapy, Ch = chemotherapy
Socio-economic groups: 1–3 = most affluent 8–10 = most deprived

- population-based treatment rates varied between health authorities for all modalities, including those forms of treatment most likely to be radical in intent;
- overall active treatment rates varied by between a third and over a half in different health authority populations.

Survival

Survival by tumour type from the date of registration is shown in Table 1.9 and in Figure 1.3. These demonstrate that survival for the clinically diagnosed group was poorer at one, two and five years than for either of the main histological types of lung cancer. The poorer prognosis of small cell in comparison to non-small cell is also shown. Overall only one in five patients were alive at a year from diagnosis, and less than 5 per cent were alive after five years.

Survival was analysed according to specialist management, using two-year survival as a marker (Table 1.10). Specialist management was associated with statistically significantly better survival in each disease category.

Table 1.11 summarises survival for different intervals using the active treatment rate of the districts of residence with appropriate statistical confidence intervals.

Table 1.9 Survival by tumour type (95 per cent C.I.): 1986–1994

Type	Survival % 1-year	2-year	5-year
Confirmed small cell	17.0 (15.5–18.4)	4.3 (3.5–5.1)	1.8 (1.2–2.3)
Confirmed non-small cell	27.6 (26.8–28.4)	14.4 (13.8–15.0)	7.1 (6.6–7.5)
Clinically diagnosed	11.2 (10.5–11.9)	3.6 (3.2–4.0)	0.9 (0.6–1.1)
All lung cancer	20.9% (20.4–21.5)	9.7 % (9.3–10.1)	4.4% (4.1–4.7)

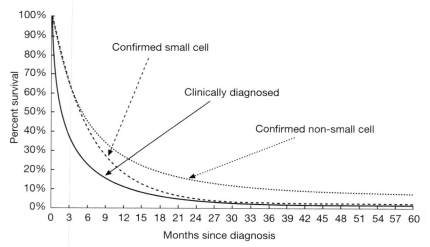

Figure 1.3 Survival of lung cancer patients by tumour type: 1986–1994

Table 1.10 Survival by specialist management: 1986–1994

Type	Specialist management	2-year survival	
Confirmed small cell	No	1.6%	(0.2–3.0)
	Yes	4.7%	(3.8–5.6)
Confirmed non-small cell	No	7.7%	(6.6–8.9)
	Yes	15.7%	(15.0–16.4)
Clinically diagnosed	No	1.6%	(1.2–2.0)
	Yes	5.6%	(4.9–6.3)

Table 1.11 District active treatment rate (ATR) and % survival by time interval: 1986–1994

Group	Survival Time (mths)	District active treatment rate (ATR) and % survival (95% CL)			
		ATR<43%	ATR=43–48%	ATR=49–54%	ATR=55%+
All	6	35 (34–36)	37 (35–39)	38 (36–39)	41 (40–42)
lung	12	19 (17–20)	20 (18–21)	21 (20–22)	23 (22–24)
cancer	18	12 (11–13)	12 (11–13)	14 (13–15)	14 (14–15)
	24	8 (8–9)	9 (8–10)	10 (10–11)	10 (10–11)
Confirmed	6	43 (41–44)	46 (43–48)	47 (45–49)	49 (47–50)
non-small	12	24 (23–26)	26 (24–28)	29 (28–31)	29 (28–30)
cell	18	17 (15–18)	17 (15–19)	21 (19–22)	19 (18–21)
	24	13 (11–14)	13 (12–15)	16 (15–17)	15 (14–16)

Lower active treatment rates were associated with poorer survival at all intervals. Broadly it can be seen that the two higher active treatment groups had a statistically better survival than the two lower active treatment groups. Whilst these differences are modest in absolute terms they indicate an important potential opportunity to improve outcomes for a substantial minority of patients in a disease in which these are poor for most patients.

The full report of this study (Cancer Outcomes Monitoring 1999) shows that socio-economic differences in survival at two years are small and not statistically different for the various super-profile groups for both small cell and non-small cell disease. For the clinically diagnosed group there is more of a gradient in outcome with the lowest three groups appearing to have poorer survival than the other groups. However this effect failed to reach statistical significance for any individual super-profile group. There was substantial variation in district of residence one and two year survival rates (not shown), but the individual confidence intervals were wide and hence these differences were only statistically significant for the worst one or two districts for each disease type. There was no consistency in the identity of these 'poor' outliers as between non-small cell and small cell lung cancer.

The full multiple regression analysis is also given in the published report (Cancer Outcomes Monitoring 1999) but one of the most important conclusions was in relationship to specialist management. The multivariate relative risk analysis shows survival comparisons made by Cox's proportional hazard regression. For each histological type, age, period of diagnosis, treatment and hospital centre were entered into the model. The results are presented as relative risk estimates, compared to a base category (value 1.00). Estimates are presented for each factor separately (sex, age, disease extent, etc); for each factor allowing for case mix (sex, age, disease extent, socio-economic status, time period, and for district standardised mortality ratio (which allows for district variability in co-morbidity)); and for all factors together, including treatment and managing specialist.

Table 1.12 shows the result of analysing specialist management of both small cell and non-small cell lung cancer within a multiple regression model. Univariate analyses are shown in the first results column, headed 'factors alone'. This shows that specialist management is highly significant in reducing the relative risk (small cell 0.31, CI 0.27-0.35 and non-small cell 0.36, CI 0.34-0.38) compared with non-specialist management. Adjustment of this univariate analysis for the case mix variables in the regression model is shown in the second results column, headed 'case mix adjusted'. This did not substantively modify the above findings. The final column headed 'all factors together' contains the mutual adjustment for all of the considered factors (a combination of the case mix factors and differences in treatment received). Again this did not have any additional impact on the results except that the scale of the relative risk reduction is now somewhat smaller (small cell 0.58, CI 0.51-0.67 and non-small cell 0.68, CI 0.64-0.72). It is clear that specialist management is an important independent variable that results in better outcomes than does non-specialist management.

Table 1.12 Relative risk analysis – multiple regression 1986–1994

	Small cell lung cancer		
Total N = 2448	Factors alone	Allowing casemix and district	All factors together
Not specialist managed	1.00	1.00	1.00
Specialist managed	0.31 (0.27–0.35)	0.34 (0.30–0.39)	0.58 (0.51–0.67)
	Non-small cell lung cancer		
Total N = 12570	Factors alone	Allowing casemix and district	All factors together
Not specialist managed	1.00	1.00	1.00
Specialist managed	0.36 (0.34–0.38)	0.42 (0.40–0.45)	0.68 (0.64–0.72)

The key conclusions about survival of lung cancer patients are therefore:

- survival for the clinically diagnosed group was poorer at one, two and five years than for either of the main histological subtypes of lung cancer;
- overall active treatment rates varied between a third and over half, and survival was shown to be better for the populations receiving higher rates of active treatment than those receiving lower rates;
- patients receiving specialist management achieved much lower relative risks of death than those who were not specialist managed, and this applied to both small cell and non-small cell lung cancer.

Overall conclusions

An important conclusion from this cancer registry-based study is that specialist management is associated with better outcomes than management by non-specialists. These data provide support for the basic premise underlying the Calman/Hine policy that patients do better if they have access to specialists in their form of cancer. Whilst this has previously been shown for some cancers such as breast cancer (Gillis & Hole 1996) and ovarian cancer (Junor et al. 1994), it is important to show to what extent it is equally true for other sites of cancer. The data from the referral study showed that an important minority of patients did not obtain access to specialists.

The widespread variations in patterns of treatment for lung cancer were substantial in the period covered by these analyses (1986–1994). This study provides some evidence that those populations receiving more active management of their lung cancers had improved survival.

Of concern is the rapid fall off in histological confirmation and active treatment with age, whatever the form of presentation, and whatever diagnostic category is used. This mirrors findings for other cancers (Turner et al. 1999). There is no evidence in these studies as to whether this is a simple reflection of general fitness, comorbidity, or frailty or alternatively whether it also includes some element of age-related practice, whether implicit or explicit. The significant differences between the management of the different age groups warrants closer examination.

If the implementation of national cancer policy, and in particular the recommendations of the National Cancer Guidance (Department of Health 1998) are effective, then the significant treatment variations described in this paper ought to reduce over time. These variations appear to be in conflict with the stated policy aim of consistent access to high quality services.

References

British Thoracic Society (1998). British Thoracic Society recommendations to respiratory physicians for organising the care of patients with lung cancer. *Thorax* **53**, S1–8

Brown PJB & Batey PWJ (1994). *Design and Construction of Geodemographic Targeting System: Super Profiles 1994. Working Party 40.* Liverpool: Urban Research and Policy Evaluation Regional Research Laboratory

Cancer Outcomes Monitoring (1999). *Cancer Treatment Policies and Their Effects on Survival: Lung. Key Sites Study 2.* Yorkshire: NYCRIS

Cancer Outcomes Monitoring (2000). *Lung Cancer Referral Patterns: The Yorkshire Experience.* Yorkshire: NYCRIS

Department of Health (1998). *Improving Outcomes in Lung Cancer.* DoH Manual 97CC122 and Research Evidence 97CC123.London: HM Stationary Office

Department of Health (1995). *Policy Framework for Commissioning Cancer Services: a Report by the Expert Advisory Group on Cancer to the Chief Medical Officers of England and Wales.* London: HM Stationary Office

Department of Health (2000). *Referral Guidelines for Suspected Cancer.* London: HM Stationary Office

Gillis CR & Hole DJ (1996). Survival outcome of care by specialist surgeons in breast cancer: a study of 3786 patients in the west of Scotland. *British Medical Journal* **312**, 145–48

Junor EJ, Hole DJ, Gillis CR (1994). Management of ovarian cancer: referral to a multidisciplinary team matters. *British Journal of Cancer* **70**, 363–70

Scottish Intercollegiate Guidelines Network (1998). *Management of Lung Cancer.* Edinburgh: SIGN Publication No 23

Selby P, Gillis C, Haward R (1996). Benefits from specialised cancer care. *Lancet* 1996: **348**, 313–18

Standing Medical Advisory Committee (1994). *Management of Lung Cancer: Current Clinical Practices.* (Whitehouse Report)

Turner NJ, Haward RA, Mulley GP, Selby PJ (1999). Cancer in old age: Is it inadequately investigated and treated? *British Medical Journal.* **319**, 309–12

Chapter 2

Screening for lung cancer

Tim Eisen

Introduction

Theoretically, lung cancer should be a good candidate for a screening programme. However, in many peoples' eyes screening for lung cancer has been a moribund topic for many years and was finally put to rest with the adverse results of three large, American, randomised, controlled trials. In this chapter the rationale for considering screening for lung cancer is reviewed, and the reasons why lung cancer screening has been discounted to date as an effective strategy for countering this important disease, are examined. The chapter will also show why screening for lung cancer has again become a lively and exciting topic for future development. All screening programmes must be practically as well as theoretically attractive and the latter half of the chapter deals with possible ways in which the developing technologies of recent years may help target screening programmes to individuals at particular risk of developing lung cancer.

Screening for lung cancer – background

When considering any screening programme three basic questions have to be considered. First, does the disease in question impose a sufficient burden of disease to make screening worthwhile? Second, is intervention likely to improve the outcome from the disease? Third, is the screening programme suggested a practical proposition? The first two of these questions are easy to answer in the case of lung cancer – it imposes an enormous health burden on the British population. There are approximately 40,000 new cases and 35,000 deaths from lung cancer annually in the United Kingdom (CRC Statistics 1999). The majority of these patients present with advanced disease and the treatment options have the limited goals of maintaining quality of life and, where possible, providing modestly prolonged life expectancy. Having said this, intervention can be extremely effective. If lung cancer is detected early in its clinical history whilst it is still resectable, surgery can provide five-year survival rates up to 70 per cent (Flehinger *et al.* 1992). The precise rate depends on stage at presentation. In stage IA disease with a less than 3 cm tumour with no nodal or distant metastases, five-year survival may exceed 70 per cent. At the other end of the spectrum of lung cancer which is generally considered resectable (stage IIB disease) with more advanced local tumour and lymph node involvement, five-year survival still reaches 30 per cent in the United States. Combinations of chemotherapy, radiotherapy and surgery have a developing role in the treatment of stage IIIA and even stage IIIB disease. These topics are covered elsewhere in this book. Where distant metastatic disease is present, five-year survival is unusual. These figures demonstrate that survival is strongly stage-dependent and that finding is largely due to the resectability of the lung cancer.

Whether screening is a practical proposition is a more difficult question to answer and there are a number of issues to be considered. Any screening test must be able to detect disease in the pre-clinical phase. The test must be accurate and acceptable to the patient. These issues were taken forward in three large National Cancer Institute (NCI) sponsored trials. However, the effectiveness and cost-effectiveness of screening for lung cancer were not confirmed in these trials. Many physicians and surgeons have formed their attitudes to screening based largely on these studies.

Randomised controlled trials (RCTs) of screening for lung cancer

Three large studies sponsored by the National Cancer Institute were powered to detect a 50 per cent reduction in mortality in the intervention arm compared to the control arm (Melamed *et al.* 1984; Fontana *et al.* 1986; Tockman 1986). The results of these studies are tabulated along with a large Czech study (Kubik *et al.* 1990) in Table 2.1. The Memorial Sloan Kettering and Johns Hopkins studies investigated the benefit of adding sputum cytology to a plain annual chest x-ray. Both studies found that the effectiveness of annual chest x-ray was not enhanced by the addition of sputum cytology. The third NCI-sponsored study has been considered definitive by many people. The study which, like the other studies, had over 9,000 study entrants, compared a standard recommendation for annual chest x-ray and cytology with a chest x-ray and sputum cytology every four months. There was no evidence of a reduction in lung cancer mortality in the control group, indeed lung cancer mortality appeared to be 6 per cent higher in this screened group than in the control arm.

Table 2.1 Randomised controlled trials of screening for lung cancer

Study	N	Control	Intervention	Results
MSKCC	10040	Annual CXR	Annual CXR and sputum	No benefit
Johns Hopkins	10384	Annual CXR	Annual CXR 4-monthly sputum	No benefit
Mayo	9211	Advised annual CXR	4-monthly CXR and sputum	No benefit
Czech	6364	CXR in years 4, 5 and 6	6-monthly CXR for 3 years annual CXR years 4 to 6	No benefit

Finally, the Czech study compared a standard arm in which study entrants had an annual chest x-ray in the fourth, fifth and sixth years of the study with an intervention arm in which study entrants had chest x-ray and sputum cytology every six months. Again, lung cancer mortality actually increased by 27 per cent in the experimental group amongst patients whose cancer was detected during the study.

A number of conclusions can be drawn from the results of these lung cancer screening RCTs. First, there is certainly no evidence of overall survival benefit from any of these studies. However, despite these studies being extremely large, they still only had the power to detect a 50 per cent reduction in mortality. If any of them had been positive, screening for lung cancer would have been confirmed as one of the most effective of any interventions possible in oncology. It may not be wholly surprising that this goal proved to be somewhat too challenging. There was also considerable contamination of the control groups in the study. For example, in the Mayo Clinic study, 55 per cent of patients in the control arm had a chest x-ray in the last year of the study and 75 per cent of controls had a chest x-ray in the last two years of the study. There has been very considerable debate about the findings in both the Mayo Clinic and the Czech studies of a higher lung cancer mortality in the intervention group compared to the control groups. This has been attributed to population heterogeneity being responsible for the higher lung cancer mortality in the intervention group. In large screening trials of these sorts even quite small heterogeneities in the control and intervention arms can greatly outweigh any effect that the screening programme itself may have. These arguments may be applied to other screening programmes and are discussed in some depth in the review article by Strauss (1998).

Despite the overall negative findings, several important positive findings emerged from these large studies. All of the studies confirmed significant improvements in the stage distribution and longterm survival of patients with screen-detected lung cancer when compared to the nationally applicable statistics. In the Mayo study, for example, five-year survival rates more than doubled when compared to the national average (33 per cent versus 15 per cent) (Fontana *et al.* 1986).

Other studies have been performed to investigate the benefits of possible preventative measures such as smoking cessation (multiple risk factor intervention trial, MRFIT) (Shaten *et al.* 1997), alpha-tocopherol, beta carotene cancer prevention study (ATBC) (Alpha Tocopherol Beta-Carotene Prevention Study Group 1994) and beta carotene and retinol efficacy trial (CARET) (Omenn *et al.* 1996). All of these studies showed significantly higher mortality from lung cancer in the intervention groups. There is overwhelming evidence that ten years after stopping smoking the risk of lung cancer is reduced by around 40 per cent compared to the risk in people who have continued smoking. Nevertheless, the MRFIT study appears to show that stopping smoking may increase the risk of dying of lung cancer by 15% (Shaten *et al.* 1997). These strongly counter-intuitive findings suggest that the biases inherent in this sort of study may apply just as strongly to the randomised controlled trials of screening for lung cancer as they do to the intervention studies completed so far (Strauss 1998).

A very large US study, the prostate, lung cancer, colorectal and ovarian cancer (PLCO) study will include nearly 150,000 study entrants and will have the power to detect a 10 per cent reduction in mortality. Screening will be by chest x-ray in the case of lung cancer, and this will provide interesting data as to whether there may be a smaller benefit from lung cancer screening than that which could be detected by the NCI-sponsored or Czech studies.

CT screening for lung cancer

Many technological advances have been made, particularly in the field of imaging, and these have encouraged investigators to re-examine the issue of whether screening with techniques more advanced than chest x-ray might be worthwhile. Two large Japanese studies have investigated the relative merits of screening for lung cancer by CT scan and by chest x-ray (Kaneko 1998; Sone *et al.* 1998). These studies showed that CT scanning is considerably more sensitive than chest x-ray in detecting lung cancer and highlighted areas that require further investigation such as the establishment of diagnostic standards and methods.

Early lung cancer action project

The overall design and findings from the baseline screening of the early lung cancer action project (ELCAP) were published by Henschke and colleagues in 1999. This study was designed to evaluate the baseline and annual repeat screening by low radiation dose computer tomography (LD-CT) in people who were judged to be at high risk of lung cancer. The baseline findings were reported in July, 1999. In this study 1,000 smokers aged 60 or older who were fit for surgery, had no symptoms or history of cancer and who had a smoking history of at least ten pack years of cigarettes, had a structured interview, chest x-ray and low dose CT scan. When a non-calcified nodule was detected by a low dose CT scan, a standard high resolution CT scan of the lesion was recommended. If high resolution scanning showed benign calcification in a smooth nodule less than 20 mm in diameter then the nodule was deemed benign. Otherwise the lesion underwent further investigation. Where there was a nodule of 5 mm or less in diameter, follow up CT scans were performed 3, 6, 12 and 14 months later. If no growth was noted then the nodule was deemed benign. If the lesion was between 6 and 10 mm in diameter a biopsy was performed wherever possible. If biopsy was not possible then follow up was as described for smaller lesions. Where a nodule was larger then 11 mm, then biopsy was performed.

The key baseline findings of this study were that 23 per cent of patients were found to have non-calcified nodules by low dose CT scan compared with 7 per cent by chest x-ray. Just under 3 per cent of patients had a biopsy according to the ELCAP criteria. Of these 28 patients, 27 were found to have malignant disease and 23 were found to have stage 1 disease. Twenty six of the 27 patients had resectable disease. The contrast between low dose CT scanning and chest x-ray is notable. Only 7 of the

27 patients found to have malignant disease by low dose CT scanning had abnormal chest x-rays and only 4 of the 23 patients with stage 1 disease had abnormal chest x-rays. Clearly, these are very early results and it will be fascinating to see how this study develops in future years. Similar screening programmes are being considered in this country and will be co-ordinated by the United Kingdom Co-ordinating Committee on Cancer Research (UKCCCR) Lung Cancer Group.

However beneficial screening programmes by low dose CT scanning may prove to be, there will be very considerable resource implications if they are to be applied on a population basis. It will be important to target screening as far as possible to those people with a significant risk of developing lung cancer.

Targeting screening

There are several possible techniques of selecting people at particular risk of developing lung cancer. The simplest is to concentrate on those people who have significant environmental exposure, usually measured in terms of a pack year smoking history. Other environmental toxins contribute to the development of lung cancer and this is a field of active research. The Roy Castle Lung Foundation is carrying out extremely detailed work to ascertain the risk conferred by a variety of environmental toxins.

There are also several clinical- and laboratory-based techniques which might find a role in identifying predisposed individuals. These techniques include cytological immunostaining (Tockman *et al.* 1997), the detection of abnormal or tumour DNA in the blood of people to be screened (Rabbitts, personal communication) and fluorescence bronchocoscopy both to identify and treat pre-malignant bronchial epithelial dysplasia (Lam *et al.* 1998).

Another attractive way of targeting screening would be to identify those individuals genetically predisposed to develop lung cancer. Lung cancer is often cited as an example of a malignancy that is solely determined by the environment. However, in addition to smoking and other environmental agents such as asbestos and radon, there is increasing evidence for the role of genetic factors conferring an increased risk. In this section the evidence of a role for genetic factors in predisposing to lung cancer is reviewed, ways in which this predisposition may be further investigated are detailed and the methods by which this knowledge might be used to target screening for lung cancer are outlined.

It is clear that individuals differ in their susceptibility to environmental insults since not all smokers get lung cancer. The evidence for this arises from studies on families with a history of lung cancer, case control and cohort studies, identification of genetic polymorphisms and cytogenetic abnormalities in patients with lung cancer. It has been known for over 30 years that lung cancer may occur in familial clusters (Brisman & Baker 1967). However, since lung cancer is a distressingly common disease and the relatives of patients with lung cancer are more likely than average to smoke, it is not possible to draw firm conclusions based on this data alone. A number of reports exist of families with a high incidence of lung cancer. Germ line mutations in the tumour suppressor gene p53 may underlie some of these syndromes (Malkin *et al.* 1990).

In case control studies a relationship between family history and risk of developing lung cancer was recognised in 1963 by Tokuhata & Lielenfeld. Over the last 20 years, 14 similar case control studies and one cohort study have been published and have shown risks ranging between 1.3 and 5.3. Eight of the 14 studies reached statistical significance. All eight studies were in western countries. Two studies in Asian populations showed no statistically significant relationship.

In segregation studies evidence was found of an interaction between genes and the environment in an analysis of 337 families with a member suffering from lung cancer (Sellers *et al.* 1994). The data were most compatible with the hypothesis that there is dominant inheritance of a rare autosomal gene which predisposed to an ealier age of onset of cancer. This means that the genetic influence is greatest in patients who develop lung cancer at an early age. It was estimated that at the age of 50, 69 per cent of lung cancers resulted from genetic factors in combination with smoking. By contrast, only 28 per cent of lung cancers occurring in patients aged 70 or older could be attributed to such an interaction.

The possible role of polymorphic variation in the enzymes responsible for drug metabolism has been examined in a number of studies. Many precarcinogens are metabolised to carcinogens and then detoxified to harmless metabolites by different enzymes. Thus, if a patient had a highly efficient polymorphism for the activation of a precarcinogen to a carcinogen, but a very weak polymorphic variant for detoxifying the carcinogen to an inactive metabolite, then it might be expected that such an individual would be at high risk of developing lung cancer. Differences in allele frequencies between patients and controls have been reported for a number of enzymes including CYP1A1 and glutathione S-transferase (Nakachi *et al.* 1993). However, the findings have not been conclusive and in any case, given the frequency of these polymorphisms, it is unlikely that any one polymorphism would impart a significant risk of lung cancer to an individual.

Several genetic loci have been identified as potential sites for genes predisposing to lung cancer. These include genes on the short arm of chromosome 3, the retinoblastoma locus on chromosome 13q and the short arm of chromosome 17. They are reviewed by Rabbitts (1994).

In summary, there is evidence to suggest that lung cancer occurs in genetically predisposed individuals. A number of leads have been identified for further identification. The obvious thing to do would be to meta-analyse the data but this is unfortunately not possible since many of the data are incompatible and the populations investigated extremely heterogeneous. For this reason it will be necessary to collect very large numbers of DNA samples and epidemiological data in order to assess genetic risk of lung cancer. Two key technological developments have made this possible. The first is the imminent completion of the human genome project which will identify polymorphisms for all 100,000 genes. The second technological development is oligonucleotide array technology which has the potential to analyse DNA sequences very rapidly and in an automated fashion. With the development of these new technologies the factor limiting further analysis is the availability of suitable DNA sample and epidemiological data collections. The Genetic Lung Cancer Predisposition Study (GELCAPS) aims to establish such a collection with DNA samples and epidemiological data from 3,000 patients with lung cancer and a group of controls. GELCAPS has the support of the UKCCCR Lung Cancer Group and the British Thoracic Society Research Committee.

Conclusion

There is as yet no proven benefit from screening for lung cancer. However, recent data from the early lung cancer action project have re-invigorated the topic and stimulated re-examination of the National Cancer Institute's three large sponsored studies for evidence that screening for lung cancer may, after all, prove beneficial. However beneficial screening for lung cancer may prove to be on an individual basis, it will have substantial resource implications. For this reason, targeting screening to those people who are particularly predisposed to develop lung cancer will be extremely important. Targeting might be achieved by several means. A combination of cytological immunostaining and genetic analysis (amongst other techniques) may allow developments in radiology to be employed to detect very early lung cancers in a susceptible population.

References _____

Alpha-Tocopherol Beta-Carotene Cancer Prevention Study Group (1994). The effect of vitamin E and beta-carotene on the incidence of lung cancer and other cancers in male smokers. *New England Journal of Medicine* **330**, 1029–1035

Brisman R & Baker RR (1967). Carcinoma of lung in four siblings. *Cancer* **20**, 2048–2053

CRC Factsheet 1.4.1998 Incidence-UK

CRC Cancerstats : Mortality – UK July 1999

Flehinger BJ, Kimmel M, Melamed MR (1992). Survival from early lung cancer: implications for screening. *Chest* **101**, 1013–1018

Fontana RS, Sanderson DR, Woolner LB (1986). Lung cancer screening: the Mayo program. *Journal of Occupational Medicine* **28**, 746–750

Henschke CI, McCauley DI, Yankelevitz DF *et al.* (1999). Early Lung Cancer Action Project: overall design and findings from baseline screening. *Lancet* **354**, 99–105

Kaneko M (1998). *CT Screening for Lung Cancer in Japan.* Proceedings of the International conference on prevention and early diagnosis of lung cancer, Varese, Italy, 9th–10th Dec 1998, pp. 144–148

Kubik A, Parkin DM, Khlat M, Erban J, Polak J, Adamec M (1990). Lack of benefit from semi-annual screening for cancer of the lung: follow-up report of a randomized controlled trial in a population of high risk males in Czechoslovakia. *International Journal of Cancer* **45**, 26–33

Lam S, Kennedy T, Unger M *et al.* (1998). Localization of bronchial intraepithelial neoplastic lesions by fluroescence bronchoscopy. *Chest* **113,** 696–702

Malkin D, Li FP, Strong LC *et al.* (1990). Germ-line mutations in a familial syndrome of breast cancer, sarcomas and other neoplasms. *Science* **250,** 1233–1238

Melamed MR, Flehinger BJ, Zaman HB, Heelan RT, Parchick WA, Martini N (1984). Screening for lung cancer: results of the Memorial Sloan-Kettering study in New York. *Chest* **86,** 44–53

Nakachi K, Imai K, Hayashi S, Kawajiri K (1993). Polymorphisms of the CYP1A1 and glutathione S-transferase genes associated with susceptibility to lung cancer in relation to cigarette dose in a Japanese population. *Cancer Research* **53,** 2994–2999

Omenn GS, Goodman GE, Thornquist MD (1996). Effects of a combination of beta-carotene and vitamin A on lung cancer and cardiovascular disease. *New England Journal of Medicine* **334,** 1150–1155

Rabbitts PH (1994). Genetic changes in the development of lung cancer. *British Medical Bulletin* **50,** 688–697

Sellers TA, Chen PL, Potter JD, Bailey-Wilson JE, Rothschild H, Elston RC (1994). Segregation analysis of smoking-associated malignancies: evidence for Mendelian inheritance. *American Journal of Medical Genetics* **52,** 308–314

Shaten BJ, Kuller LH, Kjelsberg MO *et al.* (1997). Lung cancer mortality after 16 years in MRFIT participants in intervention and usual-care groups. Multiple Risk Factor Intervention Trial. *Annals of Epidemiology* **7,** 125–136

Sone S, Takashima S, Li F *et al.* (1998). Mass screening for lung cancer with mobile spiral computed tomography scanner. *Lancet* **351,** 1242–1245

Strauss G (1998). *Lung Cancer Screening and Randomised Population Trials.* Proceedings of the International conference on prevention and early diagnosis of lung cancer, Varese, Italy, 9th-10th Dec 1998 pp. 57–97

Tockman MS (1986). Survival and mortality from lung cancer in a screened population: the Johns Hopkins study. *Chest* **89,** 324–325S

Tockman MS, Mulshine JL, Piantadosi S *et al.* (1997). Prospective detection of preclinical lung cancer: results from two studies of heterogeneous nuclear ribonucleoprotein A2/B1 overexpression. *Clinical Cancer Research* **3,** 2237–2246

Tokuhata GK & Lilienfeld AM (1963). Familial aggregation of lung cancer in humans. *Journal of the National Cancer Institute* **30,** 289–312

Chapter 3

Variations in the surgical resection rate for lung cancer: a barometer of the quality of care of lung cancer patients

Francis C Wells

Introduction

Within the current configuration of the health service in the UK there are several routes by which patients with lung cancer enter the diagnostic and treatment pathway of secondary and tertiary or specialist care. First the patient has to clear the primary care hurdle. General practitioners are over-stretched and are only rarely presented with lung cancer (once or twice per year). The differential diagnosis of patients with lung cancer is often difficult to disentangle within the primary care setting. Once the suspicion of lung cancer has been raised one of several referrals may take place, to a chest physician or chest surgeon or possibly to another specialist, e.g., a geriatrician. These various referral routes may be as a result of uncertainty, lack of knowledge about local specialist services, or preconceived ideas about the efficacy of treatment for patients with lung cancer.

The health service has been chronically underfunded. There are not enough lung cancer experts to meet demands made upon them, there is not enough equipment (radiotherapy machines or CT scanners) or experts to run the equipment, and there are not enough beds to deliver appropriate care in a timely fashion for all those who need it. The result is delays and perhaps implicit rationing at all stages.

As director of thoracic services at Papworth hospital, the author was informed a few years' ago, by the director of public health, that his purchasing authority intended to cut spending on patients with lung cancer. In particular that they would be purchasing less lung resections because, 'as everyone knew, patients with lung cancer have an awful prognosis and it is a waste of money'.

Thankfully, as a result of the ability to produce both local and international audited data, sensible negotiations were resumed. A presentation of the results of appropriately targeted surgery on properly pre-surgically staged patients, restored common sense and resulted in an increase in the number of cases purchased at a local level.

This demonstrates the worrying level of ignorance that clouds the true picture of the morbid pathology of lung cancer. The effect on outcome of treatment modalities appropriate to the stage of the patient's disease at presentation is a topic at a level of sophistication beyond many health care professionals and managers responsible for the purchase of health care. An additional problem is the nihilistic approach to lung cancer by both colleagues and the public at large.

Also demonstrated by the author's experience is the power of accurate, peer- reviewed data. The absence of such information places the negotiator in an unwinnable situation in a cash-restricted, rationed environment. It is not possible to effect change if we do not have accurate information.

Thirdly, if we do not engage in the political or managerial process, we cannot hope to change things that we may find repugnant. Mere complaining will not achieve the result we would wish to see. Constructive engagement with our political and financial masters is needed.

The ideal patient journey ought to involve the following steps. First of all, improved public education. An educated public would not smoke and would have more self-awareness of the state of their health. Secondly, although an initial screen of a patient with suspected lung cancer through a chest medicine clinic is appropriate, an adequately funded health service would allow all patients to be referred rapidly to a specialist multi-disciplinary team. However, in many parts of the UK, patients have to pass through primary and general secondary care facilities, usually with extensive delays, before entering the care provided by specialists in a tertiary care setting.

The lack of definition of care pathways that automatically lead directly to a specialist multi-disciplinary team is a major problem in many districts. The author believes that is one of the main reasons for the wide variation in resection rates across the country.

The line of referral ought to be from primary care via a chest physician to specialist lung cancer centre. Specialist units should be properly staffed with adequate numbers of thoracic radiologists, pathologists, oncologists, surgeons and specialist support nurses, in sufficient number to accommodate leave, illness and projected expansion. Of course, the patient pathway described above has now largely been enshrined within the Calman proposals. However, inadequate funding is impairing its uniform application and it is likely that the variability in resection rates is a reflection of this.

A less tangible effect of inadequate funding results in one of the greatest enemies we all face: lack of time to do our jobs properly without cutting corners. Not only is this element of our working lives dangerous for our patients, but stressful and potentially dangerous for us. Inadequate staffing, which results from inadequate funding and poor planning, also prevents those looking after patients and planning the service from having proper time for thoughtful reflection and research. This results in the low morale of everyone involved.

It is a great tribute to everyone involved in the care of patients that standards have been maintained despite the adverse conditions in which we work.

Are there any ways in which we can measure the effectiveness of the delivery of care? An important one may be the resection rate of lung cancer. Only when all potentially operable patients, irrespective of age and general condition, are seen by a multi-disciplinary team (incorporating a fully trained thoracic surgeon) can all those for whom surgery is appropriate be treated surgically. In addition, it is only in this way that those who may benefit from adjuvant therapy or down-staging chemotherapy as a prelude to resection will receive it. A process of focused specialist care will also enhance recruitment to clinical trials. If we examine the actual delivery of care we may learn something of that which needs to be changed.

Resection rates for lung cancer

Lung cancer remains the most frequent cancer in the male population. The results of treatment and the natural history of the disease remain distressing. The principal hope for our patients is that they may have resectable disease on presentation. Although little has changed in the surgical management of lung cancer over the last decade or so, the one area that has been significantly refined is the process of pre-surgical staging of the disease.

A (completely resected) stage 1, non-small cell cancer of the lung offers a possible five-year survival rate of up to 75 per cent. Therefore, in terms of potential cure, the challenge remains to diagnose the disease as early as possible and then to access expeditious surgery in specialist hands.

The UK lags behind much of western Europe and North America in resection rates. The overall figure for resection rate of lung in the UK is around 10 per cent of all those diagnosed with the disease (UK Surgical Register 1998). There are some problems in the interpretation of these data. Reference to the reported resection rates in the literature reveals different denominators in different national data sets, hence data must be interpreted with caution. However, there are some powerful messages revealed by local and regional data. In 1997, the most recent year for which data is complete, the percentage of registrations of patients in the author's region illustrates that there is a higher percentage of patients labeled as having lung cancer without histological confirmation in the regions with some of the worst resection rates (Table 3.1).

The most striking observation is the significant difference in surgical resection rates between districts across the UK. The picture in the eastern region is shown in Table 3.2. Despite similar numbers of patients with lung cancer in all districts of this region, the surgical resection rates are very different. It is this observation that led the author to formulate the hypothesis that these differences may reflect varying standards of care for patients with lung cancer.

It is also apparent that resection rates in other western countries tend to be higher than the average in the UK. Up to 20 per cent of 7,899 patients in the Rotterdam Cancer Registry underwent potentially curative resections (Damhuiss & Schutte 1996). In addition, it has recently been widely reported that the cure rates for many cancers, including lung cancer, are higher on the continent than in the UK (Coebergh

Table 3.1 Confirmation of diagnosis of lung cancer

Health districts	Registrations with histological confirmation (%)	Registration for which only data saved from death certificate was available (%)
Cambs	72.2	0.3
Norfolk	68.7	0
Suffolk	67.8	0.3
Beds.	71.9	1.8
North Essex	54.4	23.9
South Essex	55.3	19.9
East Herts.	60.8	11.8
West Herts	58.1	15.4

(Ref: Cancer Intelligence Unit, University of Cambridge)

Table 3.2 Incidence of patients treated for lung cancer 1993 and 1997

Health authorities in Oxford Anglia	Total cases of cancer	Lung cancer	Total (%)	Surgically Treated	% Surgery			
					93	95	96	97
Cambridge & Huntingdon	1995	219	11.0	22	10.0	11	14	16
East Norfolk	3339	346	10.4	40	11.6	10.25	13.7	11.3
N.W.Anglia	2108	284	13.5	12	4.2	–	–	–
Suffolk	3509	378	10.5	35	9.3	13.7	16	14
East Berks.	1838	225	12.2	16	7.1	–	–	–
West Berks.	2075	196	9.4	6	3.1	–	–	–
Bucks								
(Aylesbury)	828	94	11.4	4	4.3	–	–	–
(Wycombe)	1487	162	10.9	12	7.4	–	–	–
(Milton Keynes)	850	112	13.2	2	1.8	–	–	–
Northants								
(Kettering)	1446	117	12.2	4	2.3	–	–	–
(Northampton)	1600	182	11.4	13	7.1	–	–	–
Oxon	2890	304	10.5	12	3.9	–	–	–
Bedfordshire	–	–	–	–	–	–	12.4	12.7

Ref: Standards of Lung Cancer Care in Anglia & Oxford: Anglia & Oxford Cancer Project

et al. 1998). This data seems to support the notion that the lower rates of cancer resection in the UK may be associated with the lower rates of cancer 'cure' also reported here.

It would also appear from these data that patients within reach of organised specialist centres do better in gaining access to surgery. This observation is not simply a factor that is related to distance. It is just as likely that this 'post code rationing', is due to a lack of established lines of communication and an absence of a defined strategy for the care of patients suspected of having lung cancer.

It is likely that the establishment of a documented and agreed line of referral with clear guidelines would expedite the passage of patients through the system, and make it more likely that the optimal care can be given in a timely fashion.

In the author's experience at Papworth, where a multi-disciplinary team has existed for many years, it has been easy to reach a resection rate of 10–12 per cent. Further improvement on this was made with the introduction of a two-stop clinic with open access. This is linked to a well-defined 'hub and spoke' model of specialist chest physicians, with sessions in both the district general hospitals and the specialist centre. This has raised our resection rate to around 15–25 per cent depending on the denominator used (Laroche *et al.* 1998).

An important factor in the minds of those referring patients for treatment of lung cancer is the age of the patient. There appears to be a more nihilistic approach to more elderly patients. However, lung cancer is most common in those over the age of 60 years, with many patients over 70 and 80 years. Although advancing age adds significant co-morbidity to the outcome from surgery, it should not be a bar to surgical treatment.

Indeed, in the modern era of cardiothoracic surgery, elderly patients can perform just as well as their younger counterparts, provided they are properly selected. Hanagiri *et al.* (1999), amongst others, have shown that lung resections can be carried out safely in octogenarians. They were able to achieve a similar outcome for both the older and younger patients with appropriate selection. Indeed, this is also the experience at Papworth. The appropriate selection of elderly patients will only be made in the context of a specialist multi-disciplinary team with an experienced surgical team as an integral part of the decision-making process.

It is also important to have a culture in which all patients with local disease are considered to be operable until proven otherwise. Pre-selection of patients for surgery in the absence of an interested specialist surgeon is not appropriate.

A further important factor, which militates against the chance of a patient undergoing surgical resection is delayed referral. In 1995, the time taken from first contact with the GP to the time of surgical resection for patients at Papworth was reviewed. We found that the mean time of total delay from first presentation to GP to operation was 109 days. This wholly unacceptable delay was as a result of a multitude of factors. Delays were occurring at many different stages, with repetition of investigations frequently occurring.

The 1996 review of practice in the UK carried out by the British Thoracic Society (BTS) Standards of Care Committee revealed that this problem of delay was widespread. The average time from first chest x-ray to surgery was found to be approximately ten weeks. This did not include the frequent delay from first presentation to GP as a result of episodes of treatment for suspected chest infections and other reasons.

Whilst little data yet exists to prove beyond all reasonable doubt that delays of this magnitude will contribute significantly to a reduction in surgical resection rate, it probably does not help. It certainly causes a huge amount of stress for patients and relatives.

In an attempt to address all of the problems, we set up a two-stop lung cancer clinic was established at Papworth, in November 1995. Access was available to all GPs and physicians in the part of the region covered by the institution. This work was a Papworth initiative and pre-dated the Calman-Hine proposals. It came about from simply putting the patient first. It was then a simple matter of charting an ideal course for the patient to completion of his/her treatment. Implementation was difficult because the management plan cut across many well-established boundaries. However persistence and the clear benefit to patients enshrined in the new system allowed it to prevail. This work is covered in detail in Chapter 14.

Areas with low resection rates ought to be targeted for review of the service that is provided for patients. This bottom-up approach is much more likely to meet the true needs of the people for whom the service exists in the first place. It also clarifies the true costs that are likely to be involved. Proper planning can then ensue, and a sound strategy to ensure adequate facilities for patients can then be worked out and implemented.

The strategists and financiers should look to other examples where the customer (in this case the patient), is king and learn from mistakes made elsewhere. A more bottom-up, sensitive, listening approach is more likely to produce results.

Conclusions

Surgical resection rates can and do act as a barometer of care for patients with lung cancer. To achieve higher resection rates, approximating those of other parts of Europe and the USA, we in the UK need to examine services at a local level, and find local solutions, which must be adequately funded and resourced with the appropriate specialist staff and equipment.

References

Coebergh J, Sant M, Berrino F, Verdecchio A (1998). Survival of adult cancer patients in Europe diagnosed from 1978–1989. *The Eurocare II Study* **34**, 2137–2278

Damhuiss RAM & Schutte PR (1996). Resection rates and post-operative mortality in 7,899 patients with lung cancer. *European Respiratory Journal* **9**, 7–10

Hanagiri T, Muranaka H, Hashimoto M, Nagashima A, Yasumoto K (1999). Results of surgical treatment of lung cancer in octogenarians. *Lung Cancer* **23**, 129–133

Laroche C, Wells F, Coulden R *et al.* (1998). Improving surgical resection rate in lung cancer. *Thorax* **5**, 445–449

PART 2

Staging of lung cancer and the evidence for single and combined treatment modalities

Chapter 4

Staging lung cancer: defining the boundaries

Martin F Muers and Roderick JH Robertson

Introduction

The aim of this chapter is to summarise modern work on the classification of lung cancer and the techniques used for staging. Their role in the assessment of patients' treatment possibilities and prognosis is described. The key points are:

- staging is but one of several factors affecting prognosis and choice of treatment;
- adequate, usually cross-sectional, imaging is vital in nearly all cases;
- any improvement in the sensitivity of staging techniques may challenge present concepts of treatment strategy for example by showing that there is a bigger role for neoadjuvant chemotherapy or other systemic treatment before or after conventional surgical resections.

Staging in context

The stage of a lung cancer at presentation has a powerful influence on the prognosis and therefore the choice of treatment. However, as Table 4.1 shows, there are other factors which also influence both of these. Such factors may, in particular cases, outweigh staging information. Since the comprehensive review by Stanley (1980), many studies of these various other prognostic factors have been performed. Performance status, weight loss, histology, age, gender (O'Connell *et al.* 1986), and biochemical variables (Rawson & Peto 1990) are amongst the most consistent and powerful.

Factors which have not been so well studied include comorbidity and delays to treatment. Comorbidity is probably twice as common in lung cancer patients as in the

Table 4.1 Prognostic factors for lung cancer

Stage
Performance status
Histology
Co-morbidity
Age
Gender
Biochemistry
Treatment
Management delays

general population [Janssen-Heijgnen *et al.* 1998]. Significant comorbidity was noted in 51 per cent of the 1,600 patients with lung cancer studied prospectively by the Royal College of Physicians, Clinical Effectiveness and Evaluation Unit (1999). Recent surveys of lung cancer management in the UK have shown that there may be very long delays in the pathway of patients with lung cancer, both in primary care before diagnosis and between staging and final treatment (Billing & Wells 1996; Dische *et al.* 1996; Northern and Yorkshire Cancer Registry and Information Service (NYCRIS) 1999). Because the doubling time of lung cancer of different histologies varies widely, it is not possible to predict in a given case how much up-staging may occur as a result of delay (Geddes 1979). Delays between staging investigations and treatment may however mean that scanning data is outdated by the time treatment occurs. As a result of this, empirical recommendations have been made about the desirable maximum intervals at different points, for example, two weeks between a primary care referral and a first consultation; a week to diagnostic fibreoptic bronchoscopy; and four weeks between acceptance on to a surgical waiting list and definitive thoracotomy (Standing Medical Advisory Committee (SMAC) 1994; Scottish Intercollegiate Guidelines Network 1998).

Anatomical staging systems

Non-small cell lung cancer (NSCLC)

There is worldwide agreement that NSCLC staging should be described by using the international staging system based on the TNM classification (Mountain 1986). The most recent version of this has been published on behalf of the American Joint Committee on Cancer and the Union Internationale Contre le Cancer (Mountain 1997) (Table 4.2).

Variations include the splitting of stages I and II into A and B so that IIB includes $T_3N_0M_0$, and stage IIIA now includes $T_{1-2}N_2M_0$ and $T_3N_{1-2}M_0$.

The corresponding deductions about treatment vary a little in clinical practice, but there is fairly general agreement that stages I and II are resectable, and that, although stage III may be resectable, it should not be regarded as operable unless this is part of a multicentre trial of neoadjuvant treatment or similar. Stages IIIB and IV are generally not considered resectable. There is increasingly good survival data to support these conclusions (Table 4.3).

For example, it can be seen from Table 4.3 that the five-year survival of clinically staged IIIA patients is only 10 per cent before pathological staging and only 20 per cent afterwards. The Table also illustrates the reasonably good division in prognostic terms between the different anatomical stages and their sub-divisions.

Controversy still exists. There is doubt about the classification and outcome in cases where there are additional nodules within an ipsilateral lobe i.e., the primary tumour- bearing lobe. Presently, a nodule in the same lobe as a tumour means that it is stage T_4 and if it is in the unaffected lobe on the same side, M_1. The previous

Table 4.2 Lung cancer: TNM staging and resectability

T_1N_0	IA	}	[resectable]
T_2N_0	IB	}	[resectable]
T_1N_1	IIA	}	[resectable]
T_2N_1 T_3N_0	IIB	}	[resectable]
T_3N_1 Any $T\,N_2$	IIIA	}	[mediastinal assessment etc]
Any T_4 Any N_3	IIIB	}	[not operable]
M	IV	}	[not operable]

Table 4.3 Lung cancer: TNM staging and survival

		%					%		
		1yr	*2yr*	*5yr*			*1yr*	*2yr*	*5yr*
c	IA	90	80	60	p	IA	95	90	70
	IB	70	50	40		IB	90	80	60
c	IIA	80	50	30	p	IIA	90	70	60
	IIB	60	40	20		IIB	80	70	60
	(T_3) 60		40	20		(T_3) 80		60	40
c	IIIA	50	30	10	p	IIIA	60	40	20
c	IIIB	30	10	5					
c	IV	20	5	1					

Adapted from Mountain (1997) (with permission)
c = clinically staged; p = pathologically staged

classification was for these to be considered as increasing the T stage by 1 in the first instance and that they were T_4 tumours in the second. A recent review of 568 patients, however, has suggested that the overall survival after resection of tumours together with satellite nodules in either lobe is about 20 per cent at five years (Urschel *et al.* 1998). The author suggests that, as it is likely that the survival of patients with satellite nodules in the primary lobe alone would be better than this, and that since these lesions are resectable, a T_4 designation may not be appropriate. This discussion illustrates the general point that the staging classification is supported by very adequate evidence in general, but more data is required to clarify treatment decisions in some sub-sets of patients.

Small cell lung cancer (SCLC)

Because SCLC metastasises so readily, its prognosis is much more weakly correlated with TNM stage than NSCLC. Accordingly there is an international convention that staging should be along the limited disease/extensive disease (LD/ED) separation suggested by the Veterans Administration Lung Cancer Group (Stahel et al. 1989) (Table 4.4). Longterm survival is possible for a small proportion of LD patients but is very rare if patients are staged ED at presentation. Although the distinction between LD and ED is quite specific, there are nevertheless some differences of interpretation. For example, some authors classify any pleural effusion as extensive disease whereas others do not (Turrisi et al. 1999). It is worth emphasising again that the contribution of non-stage factors is proportionately more important than in NSCLC. The analysis by Rawson & Peto (1990) shows that performance status and biochemical variables are at least as important as the ED/LD distinction. These factors always have to be added to stage information before any treatment decision.

Staging levels

It is possible to stage lung cancer at many levels using evidence from basic clinical assessment and plain radiology, cross-sectional imaging, distant organ scanning, whole body PET scanning, via surgical staging to pathological staging by light microscopy, and then molecular analysis of superficially normal tissue to detect very small numbers of malignant cells.

Surgical survival data (Table 4.3), suggests very strongly that even conventional post-operative staging must under-stage many patients. For example, five-year survival for pT_1N_0 patients, stage IA is only 70 per cent. The only logical explanation for this is that, at surgery, there must be micro metastases without the removed lung and nodes, which cause premature death. It is this realisation that justifies trials of neoadjuvant treatments. The need for a particular level of staging investigation has to be assessed for each patient individually and the limitations of each modality have to be recognised.

Clinical staging comprises a detailed history, examination, plain radiography and routine haematology and biochemical screens. These, plus bronchoscopy or fine needle

Table 4.4 Lung cancer: two-stage system for small cell lung cancer

Limited disease	Disease confined to one hemithorax, including the involvement of ipsi and/or contralateral hilar, mediastinal, supraclavicular lymph nodes. Patients with ipsilateral pleural effusion, regardless of the type of pleural cytology, should be included in this group.
Extensive disease	Any disease staged beyond the definition of limited stage.

aspiration cytology, are basic investigations in any patient with a clinical suspicion of lung cancer. Most patients proceed to cross-sectional imaging of the thorax and upper abdomen by CT (see below). For physicians, however, an important question, when PET scanning is not widely available, is what search should be made for clinically silent distant metastases in patients who appear suitable for radical treatment.

This topic has been the subject of a comprehensive meta-analysis of 25 studies (Silvestri *et al.* 1995). Their conclusions were supported by a separate literature review (Hillers *et al.* 1994). The negative predictive value (i.e., probability of a negative full clinical examination and laboratory tests predicting a negative result on a CT (brain/abdomen)or isotope bone scan) was calculated. For the brain, the negative predictive value, NPV, (true negative clinical assessment/true negative plus false negative examinations) was 94 per cent considering six studies with 1,398 patients; for the abdomen the median NPV was 97 per cent – 1,058 patients; for bone metastases the mean NPV was 89 per cent for 633 patients, with the three largest of six studies with >100 patients having NPVs of 92 per cent, 97 per cent and 100 per cent.

Therefore, a careful negative clinical evaluation which includes no evidence of weight loss of >10 lbs (5 kg), has a probability of about 95 per cent of predicting a negative scan result.

The study included SCLC and NSCLC patients. Within NSCLC, tumour histology did not influence this conclusion, except that there was a statistically significant difference in the probability of asymptomatic brain metastases between adenocarcinoma, 12 of 104 (11.5 per cent) in four studies and squamous cell carcinoma, 1 of 47 (0.7 per cent) in four studies. Thus, for an NSCLC patient being worked up for radical treatment, there is a stronger case to be made for a routine CT brain scan if the histology of the primary lesion is adenocarcinoma. A further point to note in deciding whether to implement a policy of routine screening – not recommended by Silvestri *et al.* (1995) – is that all scans have a) a false negative rate; b) a false positive rate, which is particularly problematic in the case of bone scans (Michel *et al.* 1991). Furthermore, CT cannot easily distinguish adenomas from adrenal metastases where MRI is superior and may obviate the need for adrenal biopsy (see below).

Weight loss is commonly held to be predictive of metastatic disease, although it should probably more accurately be regarded as indicating a high whole body tumour burden. It is important nevertheless to recognise that a reported weight loss of 5 kg should lead to a vigorous search for metastases even in apparently localised disease (Geddes 1979).

Imaging staging

The role of imaging in lung cancer assessment is twofold – to give anatomical information to help predict lobectomy versus pneumonectomy, and secondly to try to stage the tumour. Radiological staging with modalities such as bone scan and CT can both overstage as well as understage tumours. To avoid overstaging, most centres will obtain tissue from enlarged nodes that are accessible and also further assess abnormal adrenal and liver lesions with MRI and, perhaps, biopsy.

Position omission tomography (PET) has the potential to answer many of these questions, but unfortunately is not widely available. A study of 100 patients with newly diagnosed lung cancer compared conventional imaging with thoracic CT, bone scanning and brain imaging (CT or MRI) against PET (Maron *et al.* 1999). The results of conventional and PET imaging were compared with pathological staging. Overall, PET was accurate in 83 per cent versus 65 per cent for conventional imaging. PET correctly indicated that 12 patients (12 per cent) were inoperable, whereas conventional imaging had considered them resectable. It correctly demonstrated as well that 11 per cent were operable that conventional imaging had overstaged. PET did overstage two and understage four patients. PET performs less well than conventional imaging at detecting brain metastases, but was better in the assessment of nodes, bone, adrenal, liver and lung for metastases.

PET scanning has been shown to be cost-effective even as an addition to conventional imaging, but more so when used to replace procedures such as bone scintigraphy (Valk *et al.* 1996). PET should be much more widely available for assessment of lung cancer patients (Scott *et al.* 1998).

Surgical staging

Surgical staging has two aspects. First, pre-resection surgical biopsy and evaluation; second, peri-operative staging. The pre-resection surgical staging procedures of mediastinoscopy and mediastinotomy are normally recommended if there is CT evidence of mediastinal lymph node enlargement to a >1cm short axis diameter (SMAC 1994; British Thoracic Society 2000). The reasons for this are first, the poor survival of patients known pre-operatively to have N_2 disease who should nevertheless have resections (Goldstraw 1992), and second, the relatively poor sensitivity and specificity of large lymph nodes on CT for neoplastic involvement. Size alone is an important but inexact determinant. The study by McLeod *et al.* (1992) showed that 13 per cent (43 of 336) nodes <1 cm short axis diameter were neoplastic, 55 per cent (14 of 57) of nodes 1–1.9 cm were neoplastic and 67 per cent (15 of 21) nodes >2 cm were neoplastic. The sensitivity and specificity of CT may vary from country to country (Armstrong 1994) but, nevertheless, surgical sampling of enlarged or equivocal nodes is international standard practice (White *et al.* 1994). Video-assisted thoracic surgery (VATS) can be used to access the pleura and chest wall and to sample mediastinal nodes, particularly those inaccessible at mediastinoscopy, but it is not as yet widely practised for this purpose. It is unlikely that the more widespread use of VATS will up-stage many patients or preclude many proceeding to thoracotomy. What is clear, however, is that the widespread introduction of guidelines relating to mediastinal sampling should reduce the number of useless thoracotomies.

Transbronchial needle aspiration biopsy (TBNA)

It is possible to perform fine needle aspiration (FNA) on enlarged mediastinal nodes (N_2) by means of transbronchial needle aspiration at fibreoptic bronchoscopy (Wang & Terry 1983; Schenk *et al.* 1987). The technique is difficult however, and not widely used. Negative samples need confirmation by open sampling and most surgeons now advise mediastinal sampling and frozen section examination before proceeding, so that the staging procedure can be done together with a resection under a single anaesthetic. In some centres, however, without ready access to a surgical service, TBNA could provide support for a CT diagnosis of N_2 disease relatively non-invasively (Harrow *et al.* 1989). The nodal stations which are easy to sample are subcarinal and the right paratracheal nodes; the others are much more difficult. As a result of this, the technique has only limited application.

Pathological staging

To date, routine standard section examination of a resected tumour and mediastinal nodes has provided the definitive staging material for lung cancer specimens. Up-staging from pre-operative estimates is common. Recently, with the problem of undetected micro-metastases in mind, resected mediastinal nodes have been re-examined using immunohistochemistry or genetic markers. This is in an attempt to see whether these more sensitive methods of detecting neoplastic cells in resected nodes lead to a better correlation of staging and prognosis.

Using immunohistochemistry and the marker BerEP4, Passlick *et al.* (1996) showed that 16 per cent of conventionally reported N_0 cases of NSCLC had micro-metastases – i.e., clusters of neoplastic cells <2 mm in diameter. In their study, the presence of these cells was associated with a reduced disease-free survival. By contrast however, Nicholson *et al.* (1997), using the anti keratin antibody MNF116, examined 1,447 lymph node slices from an average of five lymph node stations removed at resection in 49 patients who had been conventionally staged $pT_{1-2}N_0$. They found only three definite cases of micro-metastases. Disease relapse, however, was found at follow-up in 12 (27 per cent) of the other 46 patients. Furthermore, Chen *et al.* (1993) showed that a meticulous survey of resected nodes using conventional microscopy can also increase the percentage of involved nodes. Studying 588 nodes from 60 N_0 patients they found that 16 per cent had small clusters of neoplastic cells on re-examination. Because the frequency of relapse, as in the Nicholson series, seems to outweigh the frequency of missed nodal metastases, it may well be that longterm prognosis is better assessed by detecting cells in distant tissues such as bone marrow (Cote *et al.* 1995) or even blood (Margolis *et al.* 1990).

Presently, therefore, there is insufficient information on the prognostic implications of the detection of micro-metastases either by meticulous light microscopy or immunohistochemistry, to indicate whether these laborious procedures yield results with a large enough impact on staging and prognostic grouping to make them a required step in modern lung cancer management.

Conclusions

Anatomical staging alone does not give adequate prognostic information to guide lung cancer management and should always be seen as a component of a multifaceted assessment. Staging systems now used are robust and well supported by clinical data on outcome and should be used for all patients. Cross sectional imaging is mandatory for all patients who might be considered for radical treatment and for most other patients, with few exceptions. Surgical sampling is needed to verify mediastinal nodal spread or invasion as suggested by CT. PET scanning may avoid this but is not widely available so far. Careful and detailed clinical evaluation, if negative, may obviate the need for scanning to exclude occult metastases in potentially curable patients. Immunohistochemistry studies on resected nodes, bone marrow and even blood may reveal micro-metastases in a proportion of radically treated patients and up-stage them. However the clinical impact of these findings has not yet been fully evaluated.

Acknowledgements

The authors would like to thank Mrs Amanda Jones for her secretarial assistance and Dr Ian Sutcliffe for his advice.

References

Armstrong P (1994). Pre-operative computed tomographic scanning for staging lung cancer. *Thorax* **49**, 941–943

Billing JS & Wells FC (1996). Delays in the diagnosis and treatment of lung cancer. *Thorax* **51**, 903–6

British Thoracic Society Standards of Care Committee (in press). Guideline on fitness for surgery. *Thorax* **55**

Chen Z, Perez S, Carmack Holmes E *et al.* (1993). Frequency and distribution of occult metastases in lymph nodes of patients with non-small-cell carcinoma. *Journal of the National Cancer Institute* **85**, 493–7

Clinical Effectiveness and Evaluation Unit, Royal College of Physicians (1999). *Lung Cancer Audit.* London: Royal College of Physicians

Cote RJ, Beattie EJ, Chaiwun B (1995). Detection of occult bone marrow micrometastases in patients with operable lung carcinoma. *Annals of Surgery* **222**, 415–25

Dische S, Gibson D, Parmar M *et al.* (1996). Time course from first symptom to treatment in patients with non-small cell lung cancer referred for radiotherapy: a report by the CHART Steering Committee. *Thorax* **51**, 1262–1265

Geddes DM (1979). The natural history of lung cancer: A review based on rates of tumour growth. *British Journal of Diseases of the Chest* **73**, 1–17

Goldstraw P (1992). The practice of cardiothoracic surgeons in pre-operative staging of lung cancer. *Thorax* **47**, 1–2

Harrow EM, Oldenburg FA Jr, Lingenfelter MS, Smith AM Jr. (1989). Transbronchial needle aspiration in clinical practice: A five-year experience. *Chest* **96**, 1268–1272

Hillers TK, Sauve MF, Guyatt GH. (1994). Analysis of published studies on the detection of extra thoracic metastases in patients presumed to have operable non-small cell lung cancer. *Thorax* **49**, 14–19

Janssen-Heijnen MLG, Schipper RM, Razenberg PPA, Crommelin MA, Coebergh JWW (1998). Prevalence of co-morbidity in lung cancer patients and its relationship with treatment: a population based study. *Lung Cancer* **21**, 105–113.

Margolis ML, Desai B, Racely E, Schepart BS (1990). Frequency and clinical implications of monoclonal antibody detection of tumour-associated antigens in serum of patients with lung cancer. *American Review of Respiratory Diseases* **142**, 1059–62

Maron EM, McAdams HP, Erasmus JJ *et al.* (1999). Staging non-small cell lung cancer with whole-PET. *Radiology* **212**, 803–9

McLeod TC, Bourgouin PM, Greenberg W *et al.* (1992). Bronchogenic carcinoma: Analysis of staging in the mediastinum with CT by correlative lymph node mapping and sampling. *Radiology* **182**, 319–23

Michel F, Soler F, Soler M, Imhof E, Perruchoud AP (1991). Initial staging of non-small cell lung cancer: Value of routine radioisotope bone scanning. *Thorax* **46**, 469–73

Mountain CF (1986). The new international staging system for lung cancer. *Chest* **89**, 225s–233s

Mountain CF (1997). Revisions in the international system for staging lung cancer. *Chest* **111**, 1710–17

Nicholson AG, Graham ANJ, Pezzella F, Agneta G, Goldstraw P, Pastorino U (1997). Does the use of immunohistochemistry to identufy micrometastases provide useful information in the staging of node-negative non-small cell lung carcinomas? *Lung Cancer* **18**, 231–240

Northern and Yorkshire Cancer Registry and Information Service (1999). *Cancer Treatment Policies and their Effect on Survival: Lung.* Leeds: NYCRIS

O'Connell J, Kris M, Gralla R *et al.* (1986). Frequency and prognostic importance of pre-treatment clinical characteristics in patients with advanced non-small cell lung cancer treated with combination chemotherapy. *Journal of Clinical Oncology* **4**, 1604–1614

Passlick B, Izbicki JR, Kubuschak B, Thetter O, Pantel K (1996). Detection of disseminated lung cancer cells in lymph nodes: impact on staging and prognosis. *Annals of Thoracic Surgery* **61**, 177–83

Rawson NSB & Peto J (1990). An overview of prognostic factors in small cell lung cancer. *British Journal of Cancer* **61**, 597–604

Schenk DA, Brian CL, Bower GH, Myers DL (1987). Transbronchial needle aspiration in the diagnosis of bronchogenic carcinoma. *Chest* **92**, 83–85

Scott WJ, Sheperd J, Gambhir SS (1998). Cost effectivness of FDG-PET for staging non-small cell lung cancer: a decision analysis. *Annals of Thoracic Surgery* **66**, 1876–83

Scottish Intercollegiate Guidelines Network (1998). *Mangement of Lung Cancer: National Clinical Guideline.* Edinburgh: SIGN

Silvestri GA, Littenberg B, Colice GL (1995). The clinical evaluation for detecting metastatic lung cancer. *American Journal of Respiratory and Critical Care Medicine* **152**, 225–230

Stahel RA, Ginsberg GR, Havmann K *et al.* (1989). Staging and prognostic factors in small-cell carcinoma of the lung. Consensus report. *Lung Cancer* **5**, 119–126

Standing Medical Advisory Committee (1994). *Management of Lung Cancer: Current Clinical Practice.* London: Department of Health

Stanley KE (1980). Prognostic factors for surviving patients with inoperable lung cancer. *Journal of the National Cancer Institute* **62**, 25–32

Turrisi A, Kyungmann K, Bulm R *et al.* (1999). Twice-daily compared with once-daily thoracic radiotherapy in limited small cell lung cancer treated concurrently with cisplatin and etoposide. *New England Journal of Medicine* **340**, 265–71

Urschel JD, Urschel DM, Anderson TM, Antkowiak JG, Takita H (1998). Prognostic implications of pulmonary satellite nodules: Are the 1997 staging revisions appropriate? *Lung Cancer* **21**, 83–87

Valk PE, Punds TR, Tasar RD *et al.* (1996). Cost effectiveness of PET imaging in clinical oncology. *Nuclear Medicine and Biology* **23,** 737–43

Wang KP & Terry PB (1983). Transbronchial needle aspiration in the diagnosis and staging of bronchogenic carcinoma. *American Review of Respiratory Diseases* **127,** 344–347

White PG, Adams H, Crane MD, Butchart EG (1994). Pre-operative staging of carcinoma of the bronchus: Can computed tomographic scanning reliably identify stage III tumours? *Thorax* **49,** 951–957

Chapter 5

The evidence base for surgical intervention in lung cancer

John G Edwards and David A Waller

Introduction

Surgical resection for non-small cell lung cancer (NSCLC) is regarded as the only treatment that offers any hope of cure. Despite its widespread acceptance, there have been few randomised trials comparing surgery with other modalities. An early randomised trial demonstrated better survival in patients undergoing surgical resection than radiotherapy (Morrison *et al.* 1963), and in an observational study of stage I NSCLC, five-year survival for patients who underwent surgery was 70 per cent, compared with 10 per cent for patients who did not (Flehinger *et al.* 1992). Overall median survival in a group of patients who were staged clinically, but did not receive resection or any other cancer therapy, was nine months with no five-year survivors (Vrdoljak *et al.* 1994).

The decision of whether to operate on a patient with lung cancer is based on an assessment of both 'resectability' and 'operability' (Anonymous, 1997). The former relates to the *stage* of the tumour and the latter the *fitness for surgery* of the patient. The evidence base for statements of resectability and operability will be considered.

Resectability

Staging

NSCLC is staged according to the size and relations of the tumour and the presence of nodal or distant metastases. The International Staging System For Lung Cancer has recently been revised (Mountain 1997). Stage I and II were each subdivided into A and B. T3N0M0 tumours were reclassified from stage IIIA to IIB on the basis of a similar five-year survival to T2N1 tumours. Satellite nodules confined to the same lobe as the primary tumour were designated as T4 (and hence stage IIIB) in the absence of distant metastasis, whereas those in other ipsilateral lobes became M1. However, there remain clinical situations where the evidence for surgical intervention, on the basis of tumour stage, is conflicting.

T3 (chest wall) versus T3 (mediastinal)

In the 1986 international staging system (Mountain 1986), all cases with either T3 or N2 were designated as stage IIIA. However, evidence suggesting that T3N0 cases survived longer than T1-3N2 cases (Mountain 1990; Watanabe *et al.* 1991b; Green & Lilenbaum 1994) prompted the reclassification of the former to stage IIB. The average five-year survival for T3N0 tumours has been reported as 42 per cent, compared to 19 per cent for T3N1. Furthermore, complete resection confers a five-year survival in excess of 50 per cent in T3N0 chest wall cases (McCaughan *et al.* 1985; Albertucci *et al.* 1992). However, T3 tumours are a heterogeneous group: five-year survival rates due to invasion of chest wall, mediastinum and main stem bronchus and Pancoast tumours have been quoted as 33 per cent, 23 per cent, 24 per cent and 27 per cent respectively (Detterbeck & Socinski 1997). Therefore, peripheral T3 tumours (chest wall) rather than central T3 (mediastinum) tumours should be considered in stage IIB.

T4 (ipsilateral intrapulmonary metastasis)

The designation of satellite nodules within the same lobe as the primary into stage IIIB was made on the basis of survival data (Mountain 1997), which thus implies that surgical resection is inappropriate in these cases. However, there is evidence that the presence of satellite nodules within the resected lobe result in survival equivalent to stage IIIA and not to IIIB (Watanabe *et al.* 1991a). Satellite nodules in the ipsilateral non-primary lobe may represent disseminated disease and have similar survival characteristics to M1 disease (Urschel *et al.* 1998). The prolonged survival demonstrated in certain patients with synchronous ipsilateral nodules within one lobe justifies primary resection.

Surgical staging

Routine mediastinoscopy?

In a retrospective study relating the size of mediastinal nodes to the probability of malignancy, malignant nodes were no larger than benign nodes; there was a significant rate of malignancy in small nodes and larger nodes were frequently reactive (Kerr *et al.* 1992). Furthermore, selective mediastinoscopy for cases with lymphadenopathy greater than than 1.5 cm may underestimate the true pathological stage after open lymph node dissection (Fernando & Goldstraw 1990), as the incidence of unexpectedly positive N2 nodes at thoracotomy may be as high as 25 per cent (Goldstraw *et al.* 1994). Those patients with involved N2 nodes at a single nodal station may survive longer than those with more extensive nodal involvement (Goldstraw *et al.* 1994). However, the only randomised trial found that routine mediastinoscopy was not superior to a selective approach guided by CT scan in the rate of thoracotomy without cure (Canadian Lung Oncology Group 1995). Therefore, selective mediastinoscopy based on CT assessment is advised.

Video assisted thoracoscopic surgery (VATS)

VATS is also of complementary value in the surgical staging of lung cancer. This approach allows biopsy of N2 or contralateral N3 nodes not accessible by cervical mediastinoscopy and assessment of the T stage of the tumour in cases of radiological difficulty (Waller *et al.* 1997; Van Schil 1999).

Intraoperative nodal staging

It has been suggested that the incidence of N2 metastases amongst T1 squamous cell carcinomas is low enough to justify omitting intraoperative mediastinal lymphadenectomy (Asamura *et al.* 1996). However, others have found involved N2 nodes in about 10 per cent in such cases, supporting routine N2 dissection (Graham *et al.* 1999). On this evidence, the International Association for the Study of Lung Cancer has proposed the adoption of the term 'systematic nodal dissection' for the dissection and examination of lobar, hilar and mediastinal lymph nodes in a systematic fashion (Goldstraw 1997). The impact of systematic mediastinal lymphadenectomy on survival requires careful analysis. A randomised trial found that this technique was associated with significantly longer, relapse-free survival although the increase in overall survival narrowly missed statistical significance (Izbicki *et al.* 1998). However all this technique achieves is more accurate staging, which leads to greater stage specific survival.

Surgery for early stage disease

Surgical excision versus radiotherapy in NSCLC

One early randomised trial has compared the results of radiotherapy versus surgery in resectable NSCLC. A survival benefit was observed for patients treated surgically (Deeley & Cleland 1963). Radiotherapy techniques have improved considerably since then, however. Observational studies have shown survival rates inferior to surgery in patients who were medically inoperable or who declined surgery, in whom five-year survival rates of 15–30 per cent for clinical stage I patients have been reported (Haffty *et al.* 1988; Noordijk *et al.* 1988; Slotman *et al.* 1994; Jeremic *et al.* 1997).

Sublobar resection in early stage NSCLC

A randomised, controlled trial compared segmental resection with lobectomy in patients with T1N0 tumours confirmed intraoperatively (Ginsberg & Rubinstein 1995). This demonstrated a tripling of the local recurrence rate and a 50 per cent increase in cancer-related deaths, but only a marginal increase in overall death rate with segmental resection. However, with further follow-up, the survival differences between groups lost statistical significance (Lederle 1996). Most retrospective series are confounded by the indication for sublobar resection being insufficient pulmonary reserve: inferior five-year survival following wedge resection may be a result of non-cancer related deaths (Landreneau *et al.* 1997).

Surgical excision in early SCLC

A randomised trial in the 1960s, comparing radiotherapy to surgery, found that surgery was associated with a worse prognosis (Fox & Scadding 1973). Subsequently, however, the role of surgery in limited stage SCLC has been re-examined. A Lung Cancer Study Group randomised trial demonstrated no additional survival for surgery following response to chemotherapy (Lad *et al.* 1994), but this trial excluded patients with stage I tumours. Survival rates of surgically resected stage I SCLC are similar to those for NSCLC (Shepherd *et al.* 1991) – five-year survival rates of 50–70 per cent have been reported (Ichinose *et al.* 1992; Rea *et al.* 1998). Local recurrence rates may be reduced in stage I SCLC by surgical excision (Shepherd *et al.* 1991; Ichinose *et al.* 1992). The stage-specific indications for surgery apparent in SCLC support the use of TNM staging rather than the classic definition of limited or extensive disease. Classically, SCLC has been staged according to the confinement of disease to a single radiotherapy field (Osterlind *et al.* 1983). These definitions of 'limited' and 'extensive' disease in SCLC have been challenged since Shields first reported significant differences in survival according to the TNM system (Shields *et al.* 1982). However, although there are significant differences in pathological stage, there may still be differences between groups as determined by the clinical stage (Shepherd *et al.* 1991).

An aggressive interventional approach in suspected early lung cancer

Traditional management has employed an expectant policy for indeterminate solitary pulmonary nodules (ISPN), in which bronchoscopy and/or CT guided biopsy is negative but there remains radiological suspicion of malignancy. VATS has been shown to have a beneficial role in the diagnosis of ISPN (Hazelrigg *et al.* 1998). The authors have therefore adopted a policy of early VAT excision in these cases obtaining intra-operative frozen section analysis and proceeding to definitive resection under the same anaesthetic. Fifty-five patients have been managed under this protocol to date. VATS biopsy was successful in 80 per cent. There were five unnecessary open biopsies of benign lesions, but morbidity was acceptable. Overall, 67 per cent of patients had a malignant ISPN and of these, 68 per cent were stage I tumours. (Edwards *et al.* 1999a). The authors therefore advocate early excision of indeterminate ISPN.

Extended surgical resection

Chest wall invasion is an indication for reconstruction not a contraindication to excision

When tumours are adherent to the parietal pleura, extension into the chest wall is usually present. Albertucci *et al.* (1992) found that in such cases, extrapleural resection was associated with a complete resection rate of only 31 per cent, in comparison to 100 per cent if the chest wall was resected *en bloc*, and significantly reduced survival. The chest wall defects resulting from resection may be repaired with polypropylene mesh, with or without the support of methylmethacrylate cement (Hasse 1991; Shah & Goldstraw 1995). This extensive surgery is justified by typical five-year survival rates following resection of T3N0 chest wall of 35–50 per cent (McCaughan *et al.* 1985; Shah & Goldstraw 1995; (Detterbeck & Socinski 1997; Downey *et al.* 1999).

Similarly resection of tumours of the superior pulmonary sulcus (Pancoast tumours) is justified, providing previously outlined stage considerations are satisfied.

Induction radiotherapy followed by surgical resection may yield the optimum five year survival rates of 25–50 % but the role of induction chemoradiotherapy is currently under investigation (Dartevelle *et al.* 1993) (Muscolino *et al.* 1997) (Johnson & Goldberg, 1997). Extended resection (of T4 tumours) including vertebrectomy and spinal reconstruction is possible but is associated with a high morbidity and limited survival (York *et al.* 1999).

Stage IIIA disease

Neoadjuvant chemotherapy may improve post-operative survival

There is increasing evidence that combined modality therapy should be preferred to surgery alone in patients with N2 disease. Theoretical advantages of neoadjuvant chemotherapy include downstaging to facilitate local control by surgery and early treatment of micrometastases. Significant survival benefits were seen in early trials of neoadjuvant chemotherapy in a multimodality setting (Pass *et al.* 1992; (Rosell *et al.* 1994; Roth *et al.* 1994) although there has been criticism that imbalance of biological prognostic variables in the small sample sizes may have led to bias of the results (Strauss 1999). Larger phase III trials are underway. Despite the evidence to support the use of neoadjuvant chemotherapy in stage IIIA NSCLC, the role of surgery in N2 disease is less clear. There have been no randomised studies completed to compare chemotherapy or radiotherapy, alone or in combination with surgery.

Residual disease

Adjuvant therapy or re-operation?

Although the PORT meta-analysis demonstrated that post-operative radiotherapy was detrimental to survival in patients with stage I and II NSCLC (PORT Meta-analysis Trialists Group 1998), there was no influence on survival in patients with stage IIIA, N2 tumours. However, retrospective regression analysis of 224 patients at the Mayo Clinic suggested that patients with N2 nodes who are at high or intermediate risk of recurrence gain improved local control and survival following adjuvant radiotherapy (Sawyer *et al.* 1997). In the management of residual disease at the bronchial resection margin, chemoradiotherapy conferred a 14 per cent survival benefit compared with radiotherapy alone at one year (Lad, 1994). In a retrospective study, post-operative radiotherapy did not improve survival (Gebitekin *et al.* 1994). With regard to surgical re-exploration, it has been suggested as the best option for stage I or II disease (Ghiribelli *et al.* 1999), whereas it is not indicated for N2 disease.

Stage IIIB / IV disease

Surgical pleurodesis in malignant pleural effusion

Closed pleurodesis, with administration of a chemical sclerosant through an intercostal tube, is frequently unsuccessful. A wide variety of agents have been tried with variable results. Success rates using tetracycline are only 35–50 per cent and 13–70 per cent for bleomycin (Hartman *et al.* 1993; Koldsland *et al.* 1993; Banerjee *et al.* 1994; Emad & Rezaian 1996; Martinez-Moragon *et al.* 1997). Talc pleurodesis is successful in 80–95 per cent of patients (Webb *et al.* 1992; Hartman *et al.* 1993; Milanez *et al.* 1995; (Danby *et al.* 1998) and is more successful when administered by VATS than via a chest tube as a slurry. A surgical pleurodesis by parietal pleurectomy gives a lasting, effective pleurodesis (Martini *et al.* 1975) and also provides a large volume of tissue in cases of diagnostic difficulty. Parietal pleurectomy may be performed reliably by VATS (Waller *et al.* 1995). A lung entrapped by a thickened visceral cortex of tumour will not, however, be able to expand to allow pleurodesis. A pleuroperitoneal shunt may be used in this instance, (Hussain 1986) but complications, such as shunt blockage or infection, occur in up to 25 per cent of patients (Reich *et al.* 1993; Lee *et al.* 1994; Petrou *et al.* 1995). If the lung is entrapped, parietal pleurectomy alone will not expand the lung and decortication of the thickened visceral pleura is required. This may also be accomplished successfully by VATS (Waller & Rengarajan 1999).

Role of surgery in the palliation of endobronchial obstruction

Surgery has an important role in the control of symptoms due to tumours obstructing the trachea or a main or lobar bronchus which are unresectable. Options include laser resection (Moghissi *et al.* 1999b), cryotherapy (Marasso *et al.* 1998) or stents (Stohr & Bolliger 1999). There have been no randomised trials completed exploring these options: a randomised trial in the UK was recently adandoned due to poor recruitment (Moghissi *et al.* 1999a).

Isolated metastasectomy is justified In selected cases

Cerebral metastasectomy in NSCLC is rarely considered despite five year survival rates following resection of up to 45 per cent (Hankins *et al.* 1988; Read *et al.* 1989; Wronski *et al.* 1995; Saitoh *et al.* 1999). Good prognostic factors include metachronous presentation and a single metastasis (Andrews *et al.* 1996; Saitoh *et al.* 1999). Increased survival is gained from combined modality therapy than either radiotherapy (Patchell *et al.* 1990; Noordijk *et al.* 1994) or surgery (Patchell *et al.* 1998) alone.

Operability

Respiratory dysfunction

Strategies to avoid post-operative respiratory dysfunction

Bronchoplastic procedures

It is possible to preserve lung parenchyma yet still treat patients with borderline respiratory function. Sleeve lobectomy may allow complete resection of a tumour involving the upper lobar orifice or distal main bronchus thus avoiding pneumonectomy.

Operative mortality, morbidity is lower and five-year survival rates are equivalent to, or better than, pneumonectomy (Rea *et al.* 1997; Yoshino *et al.* 1997; Icard *et al.* 1999; Suen *et al.* 1999). Bronchial reconstruction is feasible even after neoadjuvant chemotherapy without an increase in mortality or anastomotic complications (Rendina *et al.* 1997). Sleeve resection of the trachea is possible in certain patients, but is associated with high operative mortality (Deslauriers *et al.* 1979; Mitchell *et al.* 1999).

VATS lobectomy

VATS lobectomy is reserved for peripheral stage I lesions and is generally contraindicated in cases of central endobronchial tumours, hilar lymphadenopathy or T3 tumours (McKenna *et al.* 1998). The apparent increased tolerance of VATS lobectomy by patients has allowed the criteria for operability to include patients at increased risk (Demmy & Curtis 1999). VATS lobectomy is safe, with mortality rates of 0–2 per cent reported in large series of patients (Lewis & Caccavale 1998; McKenna *et al.* 1998; Walker 1998) and is associated with reduced post-operative pain and hospital stay (Ohbuchi *et al.* 1998). Survival rates for VATS lobectomy are at least as good as for open surgery (Walker 1998). The possible beneficial effect on survival on VATS may be partly attributed to the reduced inflammatory response seen with VATS when compared to open surgery (Yim *et al.* 2000)

'Lobar' volume reduction surgery for cancer

The operative risk associated with poor pulmonary function may preclude surgical intervention in lung cancer. A low predictive post-operative FEV_1 (pp$oFEV_1$) is the best indicator of respiratory risk (Kearney *et al.* 1994) and a cut-off point for surgical intervention at 40 per cent predicted has been proposed. Above this level, operative mortality was zero, whereas a 50 per cent operative mortality was quoted for patients with a pp$oFEV_1$ less than 40 per cent predicted (Markos *et al.* 1989). There have been reports that the FEV_1 may not necessarily decline or may even improve following lobectomy in patients with emphysema. Korst *et al.* (1998) described a group of patients with a preoperative FEV_1 of less than 60 per cent predicted whose post-operative FEV_1 improved by 3.7 per cent. Similarly, Caretta reported a slight improvement from 69–73 per cent predicted FEV_1 in a group of emphysematous patients (Carretta *et al.* 1999). In our experience of patients with both severe heterogeneous emphysema and lung cancer who presented to our multidisciplinary team there have been 16 resectable cases with a pp$oFEV_1$ <40 per cent predicted (Edwards *et al.* 1999b). Resection was performed only of tumours situated in both poorly perfused and hyperinflated lobes. The actual post-operative FEV_1 at three months was significantly greater than the pp$oFEV_1$ (obtained by segment counting), suggesting that the physiological benefit of lung volume reduction surgery (Geddes 1999; Gelb *et al.* 1999) can be applied to lung cancer resection.

Cardiovascular disease

Combined myocardial revascularisation and lung resection

Coronary artery disease remains a significant cause of risk for patients undergoing lung resection (Detsky *et al.* 1986; Thomas *et al.* 1994). A number of retrospective analyses have considered the dilemma of coronary artery disease in a patient with resectable lung cancer. Traditionally, cardiac surgery has preceded lung cancer resection as a staged procedure. More recently, there have been concerns that the coagulopathy (Verrier & Morgan 1998) and immunosuppressive effects associated with cardiopulmonary bypass (CPB) might increase perioperative complications and cancer dissemination (Terzi *et al.* 1994; Brutel de la Riviere *et al.* 1995). This has lead to a trend towards performing both revascularisation and cancer resection under the same anaesthetic (Piehler *et al.* 1985; Miller *et al.* 1994; Rao *et al.* 1996; Danton *et al.* 1998). With the increasing interest in 'off pump'cardiac surgery (Buffolo *et al.* 1990; Ascione *et al.* 1999), simultaneous lung resection and coronary revascularization without CPB has been successful (Yellin *et al.* 1994; Hensens *et al.* 1999).

Advanced age should not preclude surgical intervention

Lung cancer is managed more conservatively in elderly patients. Data from the Yorkshire Cancer registry revealed, that compared with those under 65 years of age, almost half as many patients over the age of 75 had the diagnosis of lung cancer confirmed histologically (Turner *et al.* 1999). Patients over 75 were 2.4 times more likely not to receive definitive treatment, and their five year survival was one quarter of those under 65 years at 2 per cent. This was despite the life expectancy of 75-year-old women and men being 11.1 and 8.5 years respectively. Brown *et al. (1996)* found that, although 43 per cent of the study population in Essex were aged 75 or over, age alone appeared to account for the low active treatment rate. However, surgical intervention in appropriately selected elderly patients is justified by operative mortality rates similar to younger patients in several series (Gebitekin *et al.* 1993; Pagni *et al.* 1998; Thomas *et al.* 1998; Hanagiri *et al.* 1999). Pneumonectomy does appear to carry significant risk in elderly patients, which supports the requirement for careful assessment of operability in this group. Operative mortality is about 10–20 per cent in octogenarians (Au *et al.* 1994; Pagni *et al.* 1998). Survival figures correlate well by stage with younger patients (Pagni *et al.* 1998; Thomas *et al.* 1998) with a five- year survival rate of up to 42.6 per cent (Hanagiri *et al.* 1999).

Conclusions

The evidence base for surgical intervention in lung cancer clearly demonstrates a paucity of randomised controlled data. The majority of surgical decision making is based on Grade II and III evidence from large retrospective series. Therefore, the deficiences of published guidelines (National Health Service Executive 1998; Scottish Intercollegiate Guidelines Network 1998) should be borne in mind. However, it must be conceded that the core aspects of surgical treatment for lung cancer could not now be subjected to randomised analysis, as recruitment to the control groups would be difficult. There are areas at the limits of resectability and operability where randomised controlled evidence is needed. These include induction chemotherapy in stage II or IIIA disease and the comparative role of radiotherapy in patients with poor respiratory function (suitable only for sublobar resection) or with chest wall involvement. It is a prerequisite of the modern thoracic surgical specialist to facilitate the future search for such evidence-based practice.

References

Albertucci M, DeMeester TR, Rothberg M, Hagen JA, Santoscoy R, Smyrk TC (1992). Surgery and the management of peripheral lung tumors adherent to the parietal pleura. *Journal of Thoracic and Cardiovascular Surgery* **103**, 8–12; discussion 12–3

Andrews RJ, Gluck DS, Konchingeri RH (1996). Surgical resection of brain metastases from lung cancer. *Acta Neurochirurgica* **138**, 382–9

Anonymous. (1997). Clinical practice guidelines for the treatment of unresectable non-small-cell lung cancer. Adopted on May 16, 1997 by the American Society of Clinical Oncology. *Journal of Clinical Oncology* **15**, 2996–3018

Asamura H, Nakayama H, Kondo H, Tsuchiya R, Shimosato Y, Naruke T (1996). Lymph node involvement, recurrence, and prognosis in resected small, peripheral, non-small-cell lung carcinomas: are these carcinomas candidates for video-assisted lobectomy?. *Journal of Thoracic and Cardiovascular Surgery* **111**, 1125–34

Ascione R, Lloyd CT, Gomes WJ, Caputo M, Bryan AJ, Angelini GD (1999). Beating versus arrested heart revascularization: evaluation of myocardial function in a prospective randomized study. *European Journal of Cardio-Thoracic Surgery* **15**, 685–90

Au J, el-Oakley R, Cameron EW (1994). Pneumonectomy for bronchogenic carcinoma in the elderly. *European Journal of Cardio-Thoracic Surgery* **8**, 247–50

Banerjee AK, Willetts I, Robertson JF, Blamey RW (1994). Pleural effusion in breast cancer: a review of the Nottingham experience. *European Journal of Surgical Oncology* **20**, 33–6

Brown JS, Eraut D, Trask C, Davison AG (1996). Age and the treatment of lung cancer. *Thorax* **51**, 564–8

Brutel de la Riviere A, Knaepen P, Van Swieten H, Vanderschueren R, Ernst J, Van den Bosch J. (1995). Concomitant open heart surgery and pulmonary resection for lung cancer. *European Journal of Cardio-Thoracic Surgery*, **9**, 310–3; discussion 313–4.

Buffolo E, Andrade JC, Branco JN, Aguiar LF, Ribeiro EE, Jatene AD (1990). Myocardial revascularization without extracorporeal circulation. Seven-year experience in 593 cases. *European Journal of Cardio-Thoracic Surgery* **4**, 504–7; discussion 507–8

Canadian Lung Oncology Group. (1995). Investigation for mediastinal disease in patients with apparently operable lung cancer. Canadian Lung Oncology Group. *Annals of Thoracic Surgery* **60**, 1382–9

Carretta A, Zannini P, Puglisi A *et al.* (1999). Improvement of pulmonary function after lobectomy for non-small cell lung cancer in emphysematous patients. *European Journal of Cardiothoracic Surgery* **15**, 602–7

Danby CA, Adebonojo SA, Moritz DM (1998). Video-assisted talc pleurodesis for malignant pleural effusions utilizing local anesthesia and I.V. sedation. *Chest* **113**, 739–42

Danton MH, Anikin VA, McManus KG, McGuigan JA, Campalani G (1998). Simultaneous cardiac surgery with pulmonary resection: presentation of series and review of literature. *European Journal of Cardio-Thoracic Surgery* **13**, 667–72

Dartevelle PG, Chapelier AR, Macchiarini P *et al.* (1993). Anterior transcervical-thoracic approach for radical resection of lung tumors invading the thoracic inlet. *Journal of Thoracic and Cardiovascular Surgery* **105**, 1025–34

Deeley TJ & Cleland W (1963). The treatment of carcinoma of the bronchus: a clinical trial to compare surgery and supervoltage radiotherapy. *Lancet*, **1**, 683–4

Demmy TL & Curtis JJ (1999). Minimally invasive lobectomy directed toward frail and high-risk patients: a case-control study. *Annals of Thoracic Surgery* **68**, 194–200

Deslauriers J, Beaulieu M, Benazera A, McClish A (1979). Sleeve pneumonectomy for bronchogenic carcinoma. *Annals of Thoracic Surgery* **28**, 465–74

Detsky AS, Abrams HB, Forbath N, Scott JG, Hilliard JR (1986). Cardiac assessment for patients undergoing noncardiac surgery. A multifactorial clinical risk index. *Archives of Internal Medicine* **146**, 2131–4

Detterbeck FC & Socinski MA (1997). IIB or not IIB: the current question in staging non-small cell lung cancer. *Chest* **112**, 229–34

Downey RJ, Martini N, Rusch VW, Bains MS, Korst RJ, Ginsberg RJ (1999). Extent of chest wall invasion and survival in patients with lung cancer. *Annals of Thoracic Surgery* **68**, 188–93

Edwards JG, Rengarajan A, Muller S, Waller DA (1999a). Early Thoracoscopic Excision in the Mangaement of the Solitary Pulmonary Nodule. *Chest* **116**, 353S

Edwards JG, Rengarajan A, Waller DA (1999b). "Lobar Volume Reduction Surgery" for lung cancer: extending the resection rate in patients with severe emphysema. *Chest* **116**, A374S

Emad A & Rezaian GR (1996). Treatment of malignant pleural effusions with a combination of bleomycin and tetracycline. A comparison of bleomycin or tetracycline alone versus a combination of bleomycin and tetracycline. *Cancer* **78**, 2498–50

Fernando HC & Goldstraw P (1990). The accuracy of clinical evaluative intrathoracic staging in lung cancer as assessed by postsurgical pathologic staging. *Cancer* **65**, 2503–6

Flehinger BJ, Kimmel M, Melamed MR (1992). The effect of surgical treatment on survival from early lung cancer. Implications for screening. *Chest* **101**, 1013–8

Fox W & Scadding JG (1973). Medical Research Council comparative trial of surgery and radiotherapy for primary treatment of small-celled or oat-celled carcinoma of bronchus. Ten-year follow-up. *Lancet* **2**, 63–5

Gebhard FT, Becker HP, Gerngross H, Bruckner UB (1996). Reduced inflammatory response in minimal invasive surgery of pneumothorax. *Archives of Surgery* **131**, 1079–82

Gebitekin C, Gupta NK, Martin PG, Saunders NR, Walker DR (1993). Long-term results in the elderly following pulmonary resection for non-small cell lung carcinoma. *European Journal of Cardio-Thoracic Surgery* **7**, 653–6

Gebitekin C, Gupta NK, Satur CM *et al.* (1994). Fate of patients with residual tumour at the bronchial resection margin. *European Journal of Cardio-Thoracic Surgery* **8**, 339–42; discussion 342–4

Geddes DM (1999). Lung volume reduction surgery. *Thorax* **54 Suppl 2**, S14–8

Gelb AF, McKenna RJ Jr, Brenner M, Schein MJ, Zamel N, Fischel R (1999). Lung function 4 years after lung volume reduction surgery for emphysema. *Chest* **116**, 1608–15

Ghiribelli C, Voltolini L, Paladini P, Luzzi L, Di Bisceglie M, Gotti G (1999). Treatment and survival after lung resection for non-small cell lung cancer in patients with microscopic residual disease at the bronchial stump. *European Journal of Cardiothoracic Surgery* **16**, 555–9

Ginsberg RJ & Rubinstein LV (1995). Randomized trial of lobectomy versus limited resection for T1 N0 non-small cell lung cancer. Lung Cancer Study Group. *Annals of Thoracic Surgery* **60**, 615–22; discussion 622–3

Goldstraw P (1997). Report on the International Workshop on Intrathoracic Staging. *Lung Cancer* **18**, 107–111

Goldstraw P, Mannam GC, Kaplan DK, Michail P (1994). Surgical management of non-small-cell lung cancer with ipsilateral mediastinal node metastasis (N2 disease). *Journal of Thoracic and Cardiovascular Surgery* **107**, 19–27; discussion 27–8

Graham AN, Chan KJ, Pastorino U, Goldstraw P (1999). Systematic nodal dissection in the intrathoracic staging of patients with non-small cell lung cancer. *Journal of Thoracic and Cardiovascular Surgery* **117**, 246–51

Green MR & Lilenbaum RC (1994). stage IIIA category of non-small-cell lung cancer: a new proposal. *Journal of the National Cancer Institute* **86**, 586–8

Haffty BG, Goldberg NB, Gerstley J, Fischer DB, Peschel RE (1988). Results of radical radiation therapy in clinical stage I, technically operable non-small cell lung cancer. *Int J Radiat Oncol Biol Phys* **15**, 69–73

Hanagiri T, Muranaka H, Hashimoto M, Nagashima A, Yasumoto K (1999). Results of surgical treatment of lung cancer in octogenarians. *Lung Cancer* **23**, 129–33

Hankins JR, Miller JE, Salcman M, Ferraro F, Green DC, Attar S, McLaughlin JS (1988). Surgical management of lung cancer with solitary cerebral metastasis. *Annals of Thoracic Surgery* **46**, 24–8

Hartman DL, Gaither JM, Kesler KA, Mylet DM, Brown JW, Mathur PN (1993). Comparison of insufflated talc under thoracoscopic guidance with standard tetracycline and bleomycin pleurodesis for control of malignant pleural effusions. *Journal of Thoracic & Cardiovascular Surgery* **105**, 743–7; discussion 747–8

Hasse J (1991). Reconstruction of chest wall defects. *Thoracic & Cardiovascular Surgeon* **39**, 241–7

Hazelrigg SR, Magee MJ, Cetindag IB (1998). Video-assisted thoracic surgery for diagnosis of the solitary lung nodule. *Chest Surgery Clinics of North America* **8**, 763–74, vii

Hensens AG, Zeebregts CJ, Liem TH, Gehlmann H, Lacquet LK (1999). Concomitant coronary artery revascularization and right pneumonectomy without cardiopulmonary bypass. *Journal of Cardiovascular Surgery* **40**, 161–3

Hussain SA (1986). Pleuroperitoneal shunt in recurrent pleural effusions. *Annals of Thoracic Surgery* **41**, 609–11

Icard P, Regnard JF, Guibert L, Magdeleinat P, Jauffret B, Levasseur, P (1999). Survival and prognostic factors in patients undergoing parenchymal saving bronchoplastic operation for primary lung cancer: a series of 110 consecutive cases. *European Journal of Cardio-Thoracic Surgery* **15**, 426–32

Ichinose Y, Hara N, Ohta M, Takamori S, Kawasaki M, Hata K (1992). Comparison between resected and irradiated small cell lung cancer in patients in stages I through IIIa. *Annals of Thoracic Surgery* **53**, 95–100

Izbicki JR, Passlick B, Pantel K, Pichlmeier U, Hosch SB, Karg O, Thetter O (1998). Effectiveness of radical systematic mediastinal lymphadenectomy in patients with resectable non-small cell lung cancer: results of a prospective randomized trial. *Annals of Surgery* **227**, 138–44

Jeremic B, Shibamoto Y, Acimovic L, Milisavljevic S (1997). Hyperfractionated radiotherapy alone for clinical stage I nonsmall cell lung cancer. *Int J Radiat Oncol Biol Phys* **38**, 521–5

Johnson DE & Goldberg M (1997). Management of carcinoma of the superior pulmonary sulcus. *Oncology* **11**, 781-5; discussion 785–6

Kearney DJ, Lee TH, Reilly JJ, DeCamp MM, Sugarbaker DJ (1994). Assessment of operative risk in patients undergoing lung resection. Importance of predicted pulmonary function. *Chest* **105**, 753–9

Kerr KM, Lamb D, Wathen CG, Walker WS, Douglas NJ (1992). Pathological assessment of mediastinal lymph nodes in lung cancer: implications for non-invasive mediastinal staging. *Thorax* **47**, 337–41

Koldsland S, Svennevig JL, Lehne G, Johnson E (1993). Chemical pleurodesis in malignant pleural effusions: a randomised prospective study of mepacrine versus bleomycin. *Thorax* **48**, 790–3

Korst RJ, Ginsberg RJ, Ailawadi M *et al.* (1998). Lobectomy improves ventilatory function in selected patients with severe COPD. *Annals of Thoracic Surgery* **66**, 898–902

Lad T (1994). The comparison of CAP chemotherapy and radiotherapy to radiotherapy alone for resected lung cancer with positive margin or involved highest sampled paratracheal node (stage IIIA). LCSG 791. *Chest* **106**, 302S–306S

Lad T, Piantadosi S, Thomas P, Payne D, Ruckdeschel J, Giaccone G (1994). A prospective randomized trial to determine the benefit of surgical resection of residual disease following response of small cell lung cancer to combination chemotherapy. *Chest* **106**, 320S–323S

Landreneau RJ, Sugarbaker DJ, Mack MJ *et al.* KS (1997). Wedge resection versus lobectomy for stage I (T1 N0 M0) non-small-cell lung cancer. *Journal of Thoracic and Cardiovascular Surgery* **113**, 691–8; discussion 698–700

Lederle FA (1996). Lobectomy versus limited resection in T1 N0 lung cancer. *Annals of Thoracic Surgery* **62**, 1249–50

Lee KA, Harvey JC, Reich H, Beattie EJ (1994). Management of malignant pleural effusions with pleuroperitoneal shunting. *Journal of the American College of Surgeons* **178**, 586–8

Lewis RJ & Caccavale RJ (1998). Video-assisted thoracic surgical non-rib spreading simultaneously stapled lobectomy (VATS(n)SSL). *Seminars in Thoracic & Cardiovascular Surgery* **10**, 332–9

Marasso A, Bernardi V, Gai R *et al.* (1998). Radiofrequency resection of bronchial tumours in combination with cryotherapy: evaluation of a new technique. *Thorax* **53**, 106–9

Markos J, Mullan BP, Hillman DR *et al.* (1989). Preoperative assessment as a predictor of mortality and morbidity after lung resection. *American Review of Respiratory Disease* **139**, 902–10

Martinez-Moragon E, Aparicio J, Rogado MC, Sanchis J, Sanchis F, Gil-Suay V (1997). Pleurodesis in malignant pleural effusions: a randomized study of tetracycline versus bleomycin. *European Respiratory Journal* **10**, 2380–3

Martini N, Bains MS, Beattie EJ, Jr (1975). Indications for pleurectomy in malignant effusion. *Cancer* **35**, 734–8

McCaughan BC, Martini N, Bains MS, McCormack PM (1985). Chest wall invasion in carcinoma of the lung. Therapeutic and prognostic implications. *Journal of Thoracic and Cardiovascular Surgery* **89**, 836–41

McKenna RJ Jr, Wolf RK, Brenner M, Fischel RJ, Wurnig P (1998). Is lobectomy by video-assisted thoracic surgery an adequate cancer operation? *Annals of Thoracic Surgery* **66**, 1903–8

Milanez RC, Vargas FS, Filomeno LB *et al.* (1995). Intrapleural talc for the treatment of malignant pleural effusions secondary to breast cancer. *Cancer* **75**, 2688–92

Miller DL, Orszulak TA, Pairolero PC, Trastek VF, Schaff HV (1994). Combined operation for lung cancer and cardiac disease. *Annals of Thoracic Surgery* **58**, 989–93; discussion 993–4

Mitchell JD, Mathisen DJ, Wright CD *et al.* (1999). Clinical experience with carinal resection. *Journal of Thoracic and Cardiovascular Surgery* **117**, 39–52; discussion 52–3

Moghissi K, Bond MG, Sambrook RJ, Stephens RJ, Hopwood P, Girling DJ (1999a). Treatment of endotracheal or endobronchial obstruction by non-small cell lung cancer: lack of patients in an MRC randomized trial leaves key questions unanswered. Medical Research Council Lung Cancer Working Party. *Clinical Oncology (Royal College of Radiologists)* **11**, 179–83

Moghissi K, Dixon K, Stringer M, Freeman T, Thorpe A, Brown S (1999b). The place of bronchoscopic photodynamic therapy in advanced unresectable lung cancer: experience of 100 cases. *European Journal of Cardio-Thoracic Surgery* **15**, 1–6

Morrison R, Deeley T, Cleland W (1963). The Treatment of Carcinoma of the Bronchus: A Clinical Trial to Compare Surgery and Supervoltage Radiotherapy. *Lancet* **1**, 683–684

Mountain CF (1986). A new international staging system for lung cancer. *Chest* **89**, 225S–233S

Mountain CF (1990). Expanded possibilities for surgical treatment of lung cancer. Survival in stage IIIa disease. *Chest* **97**, 1045–51

Mountain CF (1997). Revisions in the International System for Staging Lung Cancer. *Chest* **111**, 1710–7

Muscolino G, Valente M, Andreani S (1997). Pancoast tumours: clinical assessment and long-term results of combined radiosurgical treatment. *Thorax* **52**, 284–6

Noordijk EM, v.d. Poest Clement E, Hermans J, Wever AM, Leer JW (1988). Radiotherapy as an alternative to surgery in elderly patients with resectable lung cancer. *Radiotherapy & Oncology* **13**, 83–9

Noordijk EM, Vecht CJ, Haaxma-Reiche H *et al.* (1994). The choice of treatment of single brain metastasis should be based on extracranial tumor activity and age. *International Journal of Radiation Oncology, Biology, Physics* **29**, 711–7

Ohbuchi T, Morikawa T, Takeuchi E, Kato H (1998). Lobectomy: video-assisted thoracic surgery versus posterolateral thoracotomy. *Japanese Journal of Thoracic and Cardiovascular Surgery* **46**, 519–22

Osterlind K, Ihde DC, Ettinger DS *et al.* (1983). Staging and prognostic factors in small cell carcinoma of the lung. *Cancer Treat Rep* **67**, 3–9

Pagni S, McKelvey A, Riordan C, Federico JA, Ponn RB (1998). Pulmonary resection for malignancy in the elderly: is age still a risk factor? *European Journal of Cardio-Thoracic Surgery* **14**, 40–4; discussion 44–5

Pass HI, Pogrebniak HW, Steinberg SM, Mulshine J, Minna J (1992). Randomized trial of neoadjuvant therapy for lung cancer: interim analysis. *Annals of Thoracic Surgery* **53**, 992–8

Patchell RA, Tibbs PA, Regine WF *et al.* (1998). Postoperative radiotherapy in the treatment of single metastases to the brain: a randomized trial. *Journal of the American Medical Association* **280**, 1485–9

Patchell RA, Tibbs PA, Walsh JW *et al.* (1990). A randomized trial of surgery in the treatment of single metastases to the brain. *New England Journal of Medicine* **322**, 494–500

Petrou M, Kaplan D, Goldstraw P (1995). Management of recurrent malignant pleural effusions. The complementary role talc pleurodesis and pleuroperitoneal shunting. *Cancer* **75**, 801–5

Piehler JM, Trastek VF, Pairolero PC *et al.* (1985). Concomitant cardiac and pulmonary operations. *Journal of Thoracic and Cardiovascular Surgery* **90**, 662–7

PORT Meta-analysis Trialists Group (1998). Postoperative radiotherapy in non-small-cell lung cancer: systematic review and meta-analysis of individual patient data from nine randomised controlled trials. PORT Meta-analysis Trialists Group. *Lancet* **352**, 257–63

Rao V, Todd TR, Weisel RD *et al.* (1996). Results of combined pulmonary resection and cardiac operation. *Annals of Thoracic Surgery* **62**, 342–6; discussion 346–7

Rea F, Callegaro D, Favaretto A *et al.* (1998). Long term results of surgery and chemotherapy in small cell lung cancer. *European Journal of Cardio-Thoracic Surgery* **14**, 398–402

Rea F, Loy M, Bortolotti L, Feltracco P, Fiore D, Sartori F (1997). Morbidity, mortality, and survival after bronchoplastic procedures for lung cancer. *European Journal of Cardio-Thoracic Surgery* **11**, 201–5

Read RC, Boop WC, Yoder G, Schaefer R (1989). Management of nonsmall cell lung carcinoma with solitary brain metastasis. *Journal of Thoracic and Cardiovascular Surgery* **98**, 884–90; discussion 890–1

Reich H, Beattie EJ, Harvey JC (1993). Pleuroperitoneal shunt for malignant pleural effusions: a one-year experience. *Seminars in Surgical Oncology* **9**, 160–2

Rendina EA, Venuta F, De Giacomo T, Flaishman I, Fazi P, Ricci C (1997). Safety and efficacy of bronchovascular reconstruction after induction chemotherapy for lung cancer. *Journal of Thoracic and Cardiovascular Surgery* **114**, 830–5; discussion 835–7

Rosell R, Gomez-Codina J, Camps C *et al.* (1994). A randomized trial comparing preoperative chemotherapy plus surgery with surgery alone in patients with non-small-cell lung cancer. *New England Journal of Medicine* **330**, 153–8

Roth JA, Fossella F, Komaki R *et al.* (1994). A randomized trial comparing perioperative chemotherapy and surgery with surgery alone in resectable stage IIIA non-small-cell lung cancer. *Journal of the National Cancer Institute* **86**, 673–80

Saitoh Y, Fujisawa T, Shiba M *et al.* (1999). Prognostic factors in surgical treatment of solitary brain metastasis after resection of non-small-cell lung cancer. *Lung Cancer* **24**, 99–106

Sawyer TE, Bonner JA, Gould PM *et al.* (1997). The impact of surgical adjuvant thoracic radiation therapy for patients with nonsmall cell lung carcinoma with ipsilateral mediastinal lymph node involvement. *Cancer* **80**, 1399–408

Shah SS & Goldstraw P (1995). Combined pulmonary and thoracic wall resection for stage III lung cancer. *Thorax* **50**, 782–4

Shepherd FA, Ginsberg RJ, Feld R, Evans WK, Johansen E (1991). Surgical treatment for limited small-cell lung cancer. The University of Toronto Lung Oncology Group experience. *Journal of Thoracic and Cardiovascular Surgery* **101**, 385–93

Shields TW, Higgins GA Jr, Matthews MJ, Keehn RJ (1982). Surgical resection in the management of small cell carcinoma of the lung. *Journal of Thoracic and Cardiovascular Surgery* **84**, 481–8

Slotman BJ, Njo KH, Karim AB (1994). Curative radiotherapy for technically operable stage I nonsmall cell lung cancer. *Int J Radiat Oncol Biol Phys* **29**, 33–7

Stohr S & Bolliger CT (1999). Stents in the management of malignant airway obstruction. *Monaldi Archives for Chest Disease* **54**, 264–8

Strauss GM (1999). Role of chemotherapy in stages I to III non-small cell lung cancer. *Chest* **116**, 509S–516S

Suen HC, Meyers BF Guthrie T, Pohl MS, Sundaresan S, Roper CL, Cooper JD, Patterson GA (1999). Favorable results after sleeve lobectomy or bronchoplasty for bronchial malignancies. *Annals of Thoracic Surgery* **67**, 1557–62

Terzi A, Furlan G, Magnanelli G *et al.* (1994). Lung resections concomitant to coronary artery bypass grafting. *European Journal of Cardio-Thoracic Surgery* **8**, 580–4

Thomas P, Giudicelli R, Guillen JC, Fuentes P (1994). Is lung cancer surgery justified in patients with coronary artery disease? *European Journal of Cardio-Thoracic Surgery* **8**, 287–91; discussion 292

Thomas P, Piraux M, Jacques LF, Gregoire J, Bedard P, Deslauriers J (1998). Clinical patterns and trends of outcome of elderly patients with bronchogenic carcinoma. *European Journal of Cardio-Thoracic Surgery* **13**, 266–74

Turner NJ, Haward RA, Mulley GP, Selby PJ (1999). Cancer in old age – is it inadequately investigated and treated? *British Medical Journal* **319,** 309–12

Urschel JD, Urschel DM, Anderson TM, Antkowiak JG, Takita H (1998). Prognostic implications of pulmonary satellite nodules: are the 1997 staging revisions appropriate? *Lung Cancer* **21,** 83–7; discussion 89–91

Van Schil P (1999). Role of video-assisted thoracic surgery (VATS) in staging, diagnosis and treatment of lung cancer. *Acta Chirurgica Belgica* **99,** 103–8

Verrier ED & Morgan EN (1998). Endothelial response to cardiopulmonary bypass surgery. *Annals of Thoracic Surgery* **66,** S17–9; discussion S25–8

Vrdoljak E, Mise K, Sapunar D, Rozga A, Marusic M (1994). Survival analysis of untreated patients with non-small-cell lung cancer. *Chest* **106,** 1797–800

Walker WS (1998). Video-assisted thoracic surgery (VATS) lobectomy: the Edinburgh experience. *Seminars in Thoracic and Cardiovascular Surgery* **10,** 291–9

Waller DA, Clarke S, Tsang G, Rajesh P (1997). Is there a role for video-assisted thoracoscopy in the staging of non-small cell lung cancer? *European Journal of Cardio-Thoracic Surgery* **12,** 214–7

Waller DA & Rengarajan A (1999). Visceral pleural decortication for empyema: video assisted thoracoscopy versus thoracotomy. *European Journal of Cardio-Thoracic Surgery* **16,** S124

Waller DA, Morritt GN, Forty J (1995). Video-assisted thoracoscopic pleurectomy in the management of malignant pleural effusion. *Chest* **107,** 1454–6

Watanabe Y, Shimizu J, Oda M *et al.* (1991a). Proposals regarding some deficiencies in the new international staging system for non-small cell lung cancer. *Japanese Journal of Clinical Oncology* **21,** 160–8

Watanabe Y, Shimizu J, Oda M, Hayashi Y, Watanabe S, Iwa T (1991b). Results of surgical treatment in patients with stage IIIA non-small-cell lung cancer. *Thoracic and Cardiovascular Surgeon* **39,** 44–9

Webb WR, Ozmen V, Moulder PV, Shabahang B, Breaux J (1992). Iodized talc pleurodesis for the treatment of pleural effusions. *Journal of Thoracic and Cardiovascular Surgery* **103,** 881–5; discussion 885–6

Wronski M, Arbit E, Burt M, Galicich JH (1995). Survival after surgical treatment of brain metastases from lung cancer: a follow-up study of 231 patients treated between 1976 and 1991. *Journal of Neurosurgery* **83,** 605–16

Yellin A, Moshkovitz Y, Simanski DA, Mahr R (1994). Coronary revascularization and pulmonary lobectomy without cardiopulmonary bypass. *Journal of Thoracic and Cardiovascular Surgery* **108,** 797–9

Yim APC, Wan S, Lee TW, Arifi AA (2000). VATS lobectomy reduces cytokine responses compared with convential surgery. *Annals of Thoracic Surgery* **70,** 243–7

York JE, Walsh GL, Lang FF *et al.* (1999). Combined chest wall resection with vertebrectomy and spinal reconstruction for the treatment of Pancoast tumors. *Journal of Neurosurgery* **91,** 74–80

Yoshino I, Yokoyama H, Yano T *et al.* (1997). Comparison of the surgical results of lobectomy with bronchoplasty and pneumonectomy for lung cancer. *Journal of Surgical Oncology* **64,** 32–5

Chapter 6

The evidence base for radiotherapy in lung cancer

Stephen Falk

Introduction

Radiotherapy has been used in the treatment of lung cancer for more than 50 years. In an environment where no treatment is often given for lung cancer in the UK, radiotherapy, with the intent of purely relieving symptoms, is the most commonly applied treatment. For the majority of patients, therefore, treatment that may influence survival is not given.

The principles of radiotherapy of lung cancer

The indications for radiotherapy in non-small cell lung cancer (NSCLC) are numerous and include:

- symptom palliation
- radical treatment with curative intent
- adjuvant following resection (to enhance survival)
- neo-adjuvant prior to resection.

Present research in the field is not just in optimising radiotherapy dose, fractionation and techniques, but also in exploring multi-modality therapy such as the integration of chemotherapy both prior to, and concomitant with, radiotherapy.

Palliative radiotherapy for non-small cell lung cancer

Radiotherapy can successfully relieve the major local symptoms of lung cancer. Quality of life data from patients treated in MRC randomised trials of palliative radiotherapy indicate improvement in local symptoms such as chest pain, shortness of breath and cough in more than 50 per cent of cases three months following treatment. Haemoptysis is particularly well controlled by radiotherapy in more than 90 per cent (Medical Research Council Lung Cancer Working Party (MRCLCWP) 1996). Quality of life data has also been important in indicating the high proportion of moderate or severe, often systemic, symptoms, as well as psychological distress in this group of patients often with extensive co-morbidity. Such studies have demonstrated that patients even of good functional status (WHO0-2) had a median of

11–13 moderate or severe symptoms often of a general nature, for example anxiety, insomnia, depression and fears for the future (MRCLCWP 1996). Such symptoms can also be improved by radiotherapy. Radiotherapy is also commonly employed in the management of systemic disease. Single fractions can relieve the symptoms of bone pain from bony metastases, pain or bleeding from subcutaneous or skin metastases and neurological symptoms from brain metastases.

In Europe palliative thoracic radiotherapy has commonly been given in ten treatments daily over two weeks. Such schedules are inconvenient and may represent a substantial proportion of the survival time of a patient. Long distances from patients' homes to the radiotherapy centre, possibly resulting in an in-patient stay, may also limit its applicability. Despite the widespread use of palliative radiotherapy, there are only six randomised trials addressing the questions of dose, palliative effect and survival (Simpson et al. 1985; Teo et al. 1987; MRCLCWP 1991, 1992, 1996; Rees et al. 1997). In summary, shorter schedules employing one or two fractions of radiotherapy seem to be just as efficient at obtaining symptom relief of local symptoms of lung cancer without detriment to survival time or an increase in the toxicity of therapy.

The Medical Research Council studies (1991, 1992, 1996) were amongst the first to include full quality of life data and also patient diary cards. The data generated some unexpected findings. Radiation-induced oesaphagitis is one of the most common toxicities of therapy. Whilst, as expected, one in three patients experienced such symptoms following two fractions of therapy, with a peak incidence around three weeks following completion of radiotherapy, there was no significant increase in oesophagitis following one fraction therapy (MRCLCWP 1992). Single fractions of radiotherapy to large volumes can however result in unpleasantly acute but transient chest pains and, less frequently, rigors. These acute events were not recorded in the MRC study (Devereux et al. 1997). One or two treatments have thus been widely adopted in the UK when the intent is symptom relief. The author's own practice is to limit the radiation field sizes to 10 x 10 cm for a single 10 Gy fraction to minimise the acute toxicity.

A more recent MRC-organised study (1996) asked whether or not dose intensification led to a survival advantage in patients of good performance. The results indicated that the onset of palliation was slower, but there was a small survival advantage (3 per cent at two years) with a higher dose schedule of 39 Gy in 13 treatments as opposed to 17 Gy in two treatments separated by one week. These findings were not confirmed in a similar RTOG study where no survival difference was noted between 30 Gy in ten fractions, 40 Gy in 20 fractions or 40 Gy in ten treatments (Simpson et al. 1985). Internationally now, the majority of patients with locally advanced disease and good performance status would probably be considered for chemotherapy with a view to radical radiotherapy rather than moderate dose radiotherapy as in this study. In particular, combined modality therapies have resulted in modest improvements in survival at two and five years (Schaake-Koning et al. 1992).

A further method of giving palliative radiotherapy is by endobronchial applications. This has been facilitated by the use of high-dose automated machines which can deliver treatment in an outpatient setting with treatment times of no more than 10–20 minutes. Phase II studies have shown that this can be effective in controlling the symptoms of lung cancer in up to 75 per cent of cases, and can be associated with significant improvement in airway obstruction as seen at bronchoscopy (Gollins *et al.* 1994). However, there seems to be a particular increase in the complication of fatal haemoptysis. This is usually a rare event in lung cancer occurring in no more than 1–2 per cent of patients. However, it has been reported as occurring in up to 30–50 per cent in patients previously treated by external beam radiotherapy (Gollins *et al.* 1996) and other endobronchial methods.

The Manchester randomised trial comparing endobronchial with external beam radiotherapy has, however, shown that external beam treatment provided better overall and more sustained palliation with fewer re-treatments and a modest gain in survival (Stout *et al.* 2000). Similarly, other techniques for restoring the patency of the major airways including photo-dynamic therapy, laser therapy, cryotherapy and bronchial stenting have not been compared to external beam radiotherapy in reported randomised trials. Current practice limits the wide applicability of these techniques to centres with a particular interest and the necessary equipment. In contrast, external beam radiotherapy is relatively cheap to deliver and widely available throughout the UK.

Radical radiotherapy for stage I/II non-small cell lung cancer

There are a group of patients who, although resectable, either refuse surgery or are considered inoperable because of intercurrent medical problems most commonly cardiovascular disease, general frailty, and chronic respiratory disease. Such patients can be considered for radical radiotherapy with curative intent.

There has only been one randomised control trial comparing surgery with radical radiotherapy, performed in the 1960s, in which patients were staged clinically and the number of patients treated was small (Morrison *et al.* 1963). The subsequent phase II results of radical radiotherapy are, however, extremely variable on account of differences in patient selection and methods of staging (i.e., CT versus chest x-ray) but also as a result of the extent of co-morbid disease, often tobacco-related, that characterises this patient group.

One major parameter of the success of radical radiotherapy is complete disappearance of tumour (complete response: CR) and local control. Without this there can be no long term remission or survival. CR rates range from 38–46 per cent (Zhang *et al.* 1989; Hayakawa *et al.* 1992; Rosenthal *et al.* 1992; Morita *et al.* 1997), but decline with increasing tumour volume. The best results are in tumours less than 4 cm where CR rates range from 48–52 per cent in comparison to 20–21 per cent for tumours greater than 4 cm (Krol *et al.* 1996; Slotman *et al.* 1996; Morita *et al.* 1997).

Crude survival ranges from 25–75 per cent at two years and 6–32 per cent at five years. This reflects the wide variability of entry criteria in reported studies, the majority of which are retrospective. Cause-specific survival ranges from 40–93 per cent at two years and 13–36 per cent at five years. Whilst tumour size and radiation dose appear to be prognostic variables in phase II studies, there is no consistent effect of either age or histology on survival (Clinical Oncology Information Network (COIN) Guidelines 1999). In one series there was no difference in outcome in patients who had a histological diagnosis compared to those who did not. It is therefore acceptable to treat patients without cytologically proven disease if biopsy would be hazardous, for example in the presence of underlying emphysema (Burt *et al.* 1989).

Standard US therapy is to treat both the primary tumour and the uninvolved mediastinum. However, the outcome in trials in which the mediastinum in this situation was unintentionally not included in the treatment field appear to be no worse (Krol *et al.* 1996; Slotman *et al.* 1996; Morita *et al.* 1997). This is important in a group of patients with often pre-existing underlying lung disease in whom irradiation the mediastinum increases substantially the amount of normal lung included in the radiation field and thus the potential for worsening breathlessness.

Modern treatment techniques that improve treatment accuracy using CT scanning for localisation of the disease, and conformal treatment where the shape of the radiation beam is moulded to the tumour, are generally felt to have resulted in an improvement in outcome. These techniques have not, however, been formally tested.

In summary, many patients in the UK with early stage often asymptomatic disease, and not suitable for surgery, are at present observed and palliative therapy given at symptomatic progression. The data shows that cure can be obtained in patients with low volume disease treated by radical radiotherapy and such patients should be referred for consideration of radical treatment.

Radical radiotherapy for stages IIIA/IIIB non-small cell lung cancer

Stage III non-small cell lung cancer consists of a heterogenous group of loco-regionally advanced disease. There are two subgroups, A and B, where stage IIIA disease is potentially resectable. For the majority of patients however, the disease is unresectable N2 or N3 mediastinal nodal disease or T4 disease. Here five-year survival does not exceed 5 per cent and thus treatment is usually for palliation. Without pathological staging (including techniques such as mediastinoscopy, performed in only a minority of patients treated with radical radiotherapy in the UK) it is difficult to quantify the proportion of stage IIIA and B disease. The prognosis is reported to be more favourable for stage IIIA (median survival of 12 months and a five-year survival of 15 per cent compared to stage IIIB where the respective figures are eight months and less than 5 per cent (Ihde & Minna 1991). However, for practical treatment purposes stages IIIA and B will be considered together.

Radical radiotherapy alone has been the treatment of choice for these patients on the basis that there is a non-negligible rate of complete response and a good control of symptoms (Arriagada *et al.* 1994). However there is scanty objective evidence to support this policy.

Whether conventionally fractionated (2 Gy fractions) of radical radiotherapy is appropriate at all for stage III NSCLC is contentious. Two randomised trials have shown no clinically significant advantage for immediate rather than deferred radiotherapy or between radiotherapy and a chemotherapeutic regimen without proven efficacy (single agent Vindesine) (Roswit *et al.* 1968; Johnson *et al.* 1990). When 60 Gy radical radiotherapy given by conventional 2 Gy daily fractionation was compared with single agent Vindesine by the southeastern oncology group, median five-year survivals were respectively: Vindesine alone, 10.1 months, 1 per cent; RT alone, 8.6 months, 3 per cent; Vindesine plus RT, 9.4 months, 3 per cent (Johnson *et al.* 1990). However these studies may not reasonably reflect the results of modern radiotherapy practice where staging and treatment accuracy have hopefully been considerably improved by the use of CT scanning. For example in the recent multicentre Continuous Hyperfractionated Accelerated Radiation Therapy (CHART) 38 per cent of patients were staged as N2 or N3 and 47 per cent as T3 or T4. The overall results were a median survival of 12 months in the conventional group and 16 months in the CHART group (see below).

Standard US therapy is to give 60 Gy in 30 fractions in six weeks treating both primary disease involved and uninvolved mediastinal nodes (as determined by CT scanning) in two phases. The second phase treats overt disease alone with a margin of 1–2 cm. Many UK radiotherapists treat primary recognised disease alone. There are no randomised data available. Whilst numerous randomised studies have addressed the question of radiation dose and fractionation, it is difficult to make comparisons between them as a result of variations in staging details. However, there does seem to be a dose-dependence for survival, particularly for hyperfractionated regimens (more than one treatment per day). Notably, RTOG 83-11, a study of hyperfractionation, suggested a favourable subgroup with good functional status, less than 6 per cent weight loss, and doses ≥69.6 Gy suggesting a dose-response effect (Cox *et al.* 1990).

The CHART regimen was developed in the UK. Conventionally, radical radiotherapy is given in small divided doses over approximately six weeks to reduce the longterm effects on a number of normal tissues without compromising tumour control. Tumour growth rates have, however, been shown to increase in vitro during radiotherapy. The hypothesis tested was that, by shortening the overall treatment time, the effects of tumour repopulation during the weeks of treatment might be reduced, with a concomitant improvement in local tumour control, with multiple fractions per day reducing any possible increase in late normal tissue toxicity. CHART treatment is given three times per day over 12 days including weekends in comparison with conventional regimens where therapy is delivered once daily during weekdays, usually over a period of four–six weeks. When compared with conventional fractionation the national randomised CHART study demonstrated a 10 per cent improvement in survival at two years from 20 to 30 per cent. Such results are similar to those obtained with neo-adjuvant chemotherapy. There was no significant difference in local control. Whilst acute reactions such as oesophagitis were more severe and appeared sooner in CHART-treated patients, they lasted for a shorter period and subsided as completely as did those in the conventionally-treated group. There was no increase in the late effects of radiotherapy (Saunders *et al.* 1997).

Much current clinical trial activity focuses on the integration of chemotherapy and radiotherapy. A meta-analysis of available studies undertaken by the NSCLC overview group, co-ordinated by Institut Gustave-Roussy and the Medical Research Council, used updated individual patient data from 54 randomised trials (1965–1991) and included 3,033 patients. Two distinct groups were recognised:

- older studies using longterm alkylating agent administration (665 patients) and
- modern Cisplatin-based regimens (1,780 patients).

The pooled hazard ratio (HR) overall was 0.91 (95 per cent confidence intervals 0.84–0.98, p=0.01). The HR for alkylating agents was 1.02 (CI: 0.86–1.20) indicating no benefit. However, the outcome seems to be improved by the use of Cisplatin-based regimens where the HR was 0.87 (CI: 0.79–0.96). This gave an estimated absolute benefit of 4 per cent (CI: 1–7 per cent) at two years (Non-small Cell Lung Cancer Collaborative Group 1995). The relative merits of neo-adjuvant (i.e., chemotherapy given prior to radiotherapy) and concomitant chemo-radiotherapy are discussed in the next chapter.

Post-operative radiotherapy

The use of post-operative radiotherapy (PORT) following complete resection, was previously considered standard therapy particularly following resection of N2 disease, but has been discredited by a recent meta-analysis. The results demonstrated a significant adverse effect of PORT on survival with a hazard ratio of 1.21 or 21 per cent relative increase in the risk of death. This is equivalent to an absolute detriment of 7 per cent at two years (95 per cent confidence interval 3–11 per cent) reducing overall survival from 55–48 per cent (PORT 2000). The reasons for this disadvantage are uncertain and may be due to older studies using orthovoltage radiotherapy or treatment too soon following surgery with inadequate healing. The role of radiotherapy with curative intent when resection is incomplete is uncertain. Practically it is most applicable to microscopic residual disease at the bronchial stump. The author finds residual disease at the pleural margin often impossible to localise and thus treat adequately.

Small cell lung cancer

Radiotherapy has three main roles in small cell lung cancer, all of which are discussed below.

Consolidation thoracic radiotherapy

The addition of thoracic radiotherapy reduces local relapse rates and improves overall survival when compared to chemotherapy alone in limited stage small-cell lung cancer. A meta-analysis of more than 2,100 randomised patients showed a 5.4 per cent improvement in three-year survival (Pignon *et al.* 1992). The benefit appears to be greatest for patients under the age of 55 years, and is usually to patients with limited disease and good performance status, who have achieved a complete clinical response to chemotherapy.

The timing of consolidation radiotherapy is controversial. One randomised study (Murray *et al.* 1993) showed a survival benefit and reduction in cerebral metastasis rate by employing radiotherapy concurrently with the second course of chemotherapy, consistent with previous phase II studies. Two further randomised studies have, however, failed to confirm these benefits (Perry *et al.* 1987; Work *et al.* 1997). Further phase III trials are in progress. Concomitant thoracic radiotherapy does, however, lead to increased haematological and oesophageal toxicity, and at present the COIN guidelines have therefore suggested that outside a clinical trial thoracic radiotherapy should be given after completion of chemotherapy.

Most studies have used radiation doses of the order of 40–50 Gy to the chest. In general in the radiotherapy literature there is a paucity of randomised trial data of radiation doses and techniques. Only one randomised trial addressing the issue of dose of consolidation thoracic radiotherapy has been performed. Local control was superior with a higher dose regimen of 37.5 Gy in 15 fractions when compared with 25 Gy in ten fractions (Coy *et al.* 1988). Similarly, little data exist to determine the optimum volume to be treated with radiotherapy. Often it is technically difficult to encompass pre-chemotherapy disease and the resultant volumes of lung irradiated would lead to unacceptable pulmonary toxicity. There is some evidence to support a policy of treating the residual disease and mediastinum only post-chemotherapy, which represents routine British practice at present (Kies *et al.* 1987).

Prophylactic cranial radiotherapy (PCI)

Up to 50 per cent of long term survivors with small cell lung cancer will develop brain metastases. A recent meta-analysis in patients with limited disease who obtained a clinical CR to chemotherapy has shown that PCI yielded a 5.6 per cent survival advantage at three years (Auperin *et al.* 1999). Prophylactic cranial irradiation also increased the rate of disease-free survival (relative risk of recurrence or death, 0.75; 95 per cent confidence interval, 0.65–0.86; p<0.001) and decreased the cumulative incidence of brain metastasis (relative risk, 0.46; 95 per cent confidence interval, 0.38 to 0.57; p<0.001). Whilst there was a trend for higher doses of radiation to yield greater decreases in the risk of brain metastasis, the effect on survival did not differ significantly according to the dose. There are continuing concerns about the neuro-psychiatric consequences of PCI. However, a recent randomised trial which assessed cognitive function prospectively during the study did not demonstrate enhanced risk in patients treated with cranial radiation compared to chemotherapy alone (Gregor *et al.* 1997).

Palliative radiotherapy

When chemotherapy fails palliative radiotherapy may be administered using the same fractionation and techniques as for non-small cell lung cancer.

Conclusions

For the majority of patients with regionally advanced non-small cell lung cancer and of poor functional status, palliative therapy is appropriate. Carefully selected patients with good performance status and limited bulk of disease may be treated with radical radiation therapy alone and cure is recognised. However, there is increasing evidence that in particular for more advanced disease multimodal therapy employing chemotherapy, radiotherapy and surgery in combination, in addition to novel radiation-fractionation regimens such as CHART, can improve outcomes.

For small cell lung cancer, meta-analyses have confirmed the role of radiotherapy as an adjuvant to the thorax and cranium.

The further development of radiotherapy in the UK for lung cancer must primarily be driven by the implementation of more radical treatment for appropriately selected patients (e.g., the introduction of CHART nationwide). Thus treatment is given with the intent to alter the course of the disease rather than purely for symptom relief. There will be increasing integration with other treatment modalities. Such strategies require effective multi-disciplinary team-working.

References

Arriagada R, Stewart LA, Pignon JP *et al.* (1994). Combined radio-chemotherapy in the management of locally advanced non-small cell lung cancer (NSCLC). *Lung Cancer* **11**, 146–147

Auperin A, Arriagada R, Pignon JP *et al.* (1999). Prophylactic cranial irradiation for patients with small-cell lung cancer in complete remission. Prophylactic Cranial Irradiation Overview Collaborative Group. *New England Journal of Medicine* **341**, 476–84

Burt PA, Hancock BM, Stout R (1989). Radical radiotherapy for carcinoma of the bronchus: an equal alternative to radical surgery? *Clinical Oncology* **1**, 86–90

COIN Lung Cancer Working Group (1999). Guidelines on the non-surgical management of lung cancer. *Clinical Onology* **11**, S23

Cox JD, Azarnia N, Byhardt RW *et al.* (1990). A randomized phase I/II trial of hyperfractionated radiation therapy with total doses of 60.9 Gy to 79.2 Gy: possible survival benefit with 69.6 Gy in favourable patients with Radiation Therapy Oncology Group stage III non-small cell lung carcinoma: report of Radiation Therapy Oncology Group 83-11. *Journal of Clinical Oncology* **8,** 1543–55

Coy P, Hodson I, Payne DG *et al.* (1988). The effects of dose of thoracic irradiation on recurrence in patients with limited stage small cell lung cancer: Initial results of a Canadian multicenter randomised trial. *International Journal of Radiation Oncology, Biology, Physics.* **14,** 219–226

Devereux S, Hatton MFQ, Macbeth FR (1997). Immediate side effects of large fraction radiotherapy. *Clinical Oncology* **9,** 96–99

Gollins SW, Burt PA, Barber PV, Stout R (1994). High dose rate intraluminal radiotherapy for carinoma of the bronchus: outcome of treatment of 406 patients. *Radiotherapy in Oncology* **33,** 31–40

Gollins SW, Ryder WD, Burt PA, Barber PV, Stout R (1996). Massive haemoptysis death and other morbidity associated with high dose rate intraluminal radiotherapy for carcinoma of the bronchus. *Radiotherapy in Oncology* **39,** 105–116

Gregor A, Cull A, Stephens RJ *et al.* (1997). Prophylactic cranial irradiation is indicated following complete response to induction therapy in small cell lung cancer: results of a multicentre randomised trial. *European Journal of Cancer* **33,** 1752–1758

Hyawaka K, Mituhashi N, Nakajima N *et al.* (1992). Radiation therapy for stage I-III epidermoid carcinoma of the lung. *Lung Cancer* **8,** 213–214

Ihde DC & Minna JD (1991). Non-small cell lung cancer. Part I: Biology diagnosis and staging. *Current Problems in Cancer* **15,** 63–104

Johnson DH, Einhorn LH, Bartolucci A *et al.* (1990). Thoracic radiotherapy does not prolong survival in patients with locally advanced unresectable non-small cell lung cancer. *Annals of Internal Medicine* **113,** 33–38

Kies MS, Mira JG, Crowley JJ *et al.* (1987). Multimodal therapy for limited small-cell lung cancer: A randomized study of induction chemotherapy with or without thoracic radiation in complete responders; and with wide field versus reduced-field radiation in partial responders. A Southwest Oncology Group Study. *Journal of Clinical Oncology* **5,** 592–600

Krol ADG, Aussems P, Noordijk EM, Hermans J, Leer JWH (1996). Local irradiation alone for peripheral stage I lung cancer: could we omit the elctive regional node irradiation? *International Journal of Radiation Oncology, Biology, Physics* **34,** 297–302

Medical Research Council Lung Cancer Working Party (1991). Inoperable non-small cell lung cancer (NSCLC): A Medical Research Council randomised trial of palliative radiotherapy with two fractions or ten fractions. *British Journal of Cancer* **63,** 265–271

Medical Research Council Lung Cancer Working Party (1992). A Medical Research Council randomised trial of palliative radiotherapy with two fractions or a single fraction with inoperable non-small cell lung cancer and poor performance status. *British Journal of Cancer* **65,** 934–941

Medical Research Council Lung Cancer Working Party (1996). Randomised trial of palliative two-fraction versus more intensive 13-fraction radiotherapy for patients with inoperable non-small cell lung cancer. *Clinical Oncology* **8,** 167–175

Morita K, Fuwa N, Suzuki Y *et al.* (1997). Radical radiotherapy for medically inoperable non-small cell lung cancer in clinical stage I: a retrospective analysis of 149 patients. *Radiotherapy in Oncology* **42,** 31–36

Morrison R, Deeley TJ, Cleland WP (1963). The treatment of carcinoma of the bronchus. A clinical trial to compare surgery and supervoltage radiotherapy. *Lancet* **I,** 683–684

Murray N, Coy P, Pater JL *et al.* (1993). Importance of timing for thoracic irradiation in the combined modality treatment of limited stage small cell lung cancer. *Journal of Clinical Oncology* **11,** 336–344

Non-small Cell Lung Cancer Collaborative Group (1995). Chemotherapy in non-small cell lung cancer: a meta-analysis using updated data on individual patients from 52 randomised trials. *British Medical Journal* **311,** 899–900

Perry MC, Eaton WL, Propert KJ *et al.* (1987). Chemotherapy with or without radiation therapy in limited small-cell carcinoma of the lung. *New England Journal of Medicine* **316,** 912–918

Pignon JP, Arriagada R, Ihde DC *et al.* (1992). A meta-analysis of thoracic radiotherapy for small -cell lung cancer. *New England Journal of Medicine* **327,** 1618–1624

PORT Meta-Analysis Trialists Group (2000). Postoperative radiotherapy for non-small cell lung cancer. *Cochrane Database System Review* 2:CD002142

Rees GJG, Devrell CE, Barley VL, Newman HFV (1997) Palliative radiotherapy for lung cancer: two versus five fractions. *Clinical Oncology* **9,** 90–95

Rosenthal SA, Curran WJ, Herbert SH *et al.* (1992). Clinical stage II non-small cell cancer treated with radiation therapy alone. *Cancer* **70,** 2410–2417

Roswit B, Patno ME, Rapp R *et al.* (1968). The survival of patients with inoperable lung cancer: a large-scale randomized study of radiation therapy versus placebo. *Radiology* **90,** 688–697

Saunders M, Dische S, Barrett A *et al.* (1997). Continuous hyperfractionated accelerated radiotherapy (CHART) versus conventional radiotherapy in non-small cell lung cancer: a randomised multicentre trial. *Lancet* **350,** 161–165

Schaake-Koning C, van den Bogaert W, Dalesio O *et al.* (1992). Effects of concomitant cisplatin and radiotherapy on inoperable non-small-cell lung cancer. *New England Journal of Medicine* **326,** 524–30

Simpson JR, Francis ME, Perez-Tamyo R, Marks RD, Rao DV (1985). Palliative radiotherapy for inoperable carcinoma of the lung: final report of a RTOG multi-institutional trial. *International Journal of Radiation Oncology, Biology Physics* **11,** 752–758.

Slotman BJ, Antonisse IE, Njo KH. (1996). Limited field irradiation in early stage (T1-2N0) non-small cell lung cancer. *Radiotherapy in Oncology* **41,** 41–44

Stout R, Barker P, Purt P *et al.* (2000). *Radiotherapy in Oncology* **56,** 323–27

Teo P, Tai TH, Tsui KH (1987). A randomized study on palliative radiation for inoperable non small cell carcinoma of the lung. *International Journal of Radiation Oncology, Biology, Physics* **14,** 867–871

Work E, Nielsen OS, Bentzen S M *et al.* (1997). Randomized study of initial versus late chest irradiation combined with chemotherapy in limited stage small-cell lung cancer. *Journal of Clinical Oncology* **15,** 3030–3037

Zhang HX, Yin WB, Zhang LJ *et al.* (1989). Curative radiotherapy of early operable non-small cell lung cancer. *Radiotherapy in Oncology* **14,** 89–94

Chapter 7

The evidence base for combined modality treatment in lung cancer

Anna Gregor

Introduction

Chances of survival after the diagnosis of lung cancer remain poor and in the UK have not changed over the last two decades (Janssen-Heijnen *et al.* 1998). One reason for this is the small proportion of lung cancer patients receiving curative treatment, but, even in the best surgical series, about two thirds of patients recur after apparently complete tumour resection. This is caused predominantly by systemic metastases but local recurrence in the chest or a combination of both of these events is also troublesome (Aisner *et al.* 1983). An understanding of the natural history of treated lung cancer has lead to the realisation that single modality of treatment however optimised will not be able to improve matters. This conclusion, together with developments in systemic chemotherapy and irradiation, has resulted in the adoption of combined modality treatments as the standard measurement in a variety of lung cancer settings. This strategy has resulted in improved survival for a substantial number of patients (Pignon *et al.* 1992; Non-Small Cell Lung Cancer Collaborative Group 1995). However, the magnitude of benefit in separate prognostic groups or in individual patients is modest. There are a number of issue regarding selection of patients likely to benefit, choice of treatments and optimal schedule, which remain to be resolved.

This chapter reviews the currently available evidence supporting the use of combined modality therapy in the treatment of lung cancer.

Two pivotal meta-analyses published more than five years ago (Pignon *et al.* 1992; Non-Small Cell Lung Cancer Collaborative Group 1995) were the first to be able to quantify the benefit of this combined modality treatment. Despite this evidence, recent audits show that combined modality therapy has not been widely adopted in the UK and remains the exception rather than the rule (Fergusson *et al.* 1996). The frequency of lung cancer, its poor and unchanging prognosis (Janssen-Heijnen *et al.* 1998) and the modest additional demands of combined modality treatments both in terms of toxicity and treatment costs demand an urgent review of national policy and the introduction of combined modality treatments into clinical practice.

For the purposes of further discussion the evidence is split into two groups based on the histological type of the lung cancer.

The evidence for use of combined modality treatment in patients with small cell lung cancer (SCLC)

For patients with small cell lung cancer (SCLC) the primary treatment is chemotherapy. Combined modality treatment therefore refers to the addition of thoracic irradiation (TI) and prophylactic cranial irradiation (PCI) to combination chemotherapy.

TI halves the rates of local recurrences and leads to a 14 per cent reduction in mortality (HR 0.86; 95 per cent CI 0.78–0.94; p=0.001) with an absolute three-year survival benefit of 5.4 per cent (Pignon *et al.* 1992). The benefits of TI appear to be greatest for younger patients. In patients < 55 years of age the RR was 0.72 (95 per cent CI 0.56–0.93), whilst in patients > 70 TI failed to provide benefit. TI leads to an increase in pulmonary toxicity particularly when combined with drugs such as cyclophosphomide and adriamycin (5 per cent versus 28 per cent incidence of pneumonitis).

In patients achieving remission with induction treatment (chemotherapy or chemotherapy with TI), PCI improves both overall and disease-free survival (Auperin *et al.* 1999). PCI leads to a 5.4 per cent increase in rate of survival at three years from 15.3 per cent to 20.7 per cent; HR 0.84 (95 per cent CI 0.73–0.97); p=0.01. PCI increases the rate of disease-free survival RR 0.75; (95 per cent CI 0.65–0.86); p<0.001 and decreases the cumulative incidence of brain metastases RR 0.46; (95 per cent CI 0.38–0.57); p<0.001. The beneficial effects of PCI and TI on local control rates and survival are independent of each other and may be additional with the potential of a more than 10 per cent improvement in three-year survival for appropriately treated patients. This would represent a highly significant advance in a disease setting where there has been little progress for more than a decade.

Unresolved issues, where current evidence is insufficient or conflicting and which need to be explored further in randomised trials, relate to:

* concurrent or sequential administration of TI particularly with chemotherapy agents which may have different toxicity profiles from the current standard of platinum /VP-16 combinations;
* hyperfractionation or accelerated fractionation of TI which brings increased acute toxicity to organs such as the oesophagus, as well as the possibility of improved therapeutic ratio for normal lung and higher biological effectiveness against the tumour;
* defining optimal radiation dose, schedule and timing of PCI as well as investigation of cognitive abnormalities in SCLC patients.

Some of these trials are already ongoing or planned, but patient recruitment is often slow and constrained by the current UK practice of sequential approach to chemotherapy and irradiation. Closer working relationships between respiratory physicians and medical and radiation oncologists offered by the development of clinical networks may resolve some of these problems and lead to collaborations capable of delivering sophisticated schedules of combined modality treatments to selected patients.

The evidence base for use of combined modality treatments in non small cell lung cancer (NSCLC)

For patients with other histological subtypes of lung cancer (NSCLC) the primary treatment is either surgery or TI.

Platinum-based chemotherapy leads to a 13 per cent reduction in the risk of death at two years and provides an absolute benefit of 4 per cent (95 per cent CI 1–7 per cent) at two years. At five years, an absolute benefit of 2 per cent (95 per cent CI 1–4 per cent) is seen (Non-Small Cell Lung Cancer Collaborative Group 1995). The advantage of chemotherapy has been seen in patients with all stages of disease and in all the prognostic groups examined in the overview. The magnitude of benefit is largest in patients with advanced disease where the risk reduction is 27 per cent – equivalent to an absolute survival benefit of 10 per cent (95 per cent CI 5–15 per cent) at one year.

In trials testing the issue of symptom control and quality of life (QOL) chemotherapy appears to be better than best supportive care but the evidence is not conclusive and results from future trials (e.g., the Big Lung Trial in the UK) are awaited (Ihde 1992; American Society of Clinical Oncology 1997).

The current debate centres on how best to schedule combined modality treatment in patients with NSCLC. In patients with resectable tumours, a number of large intergroup trials testing the value of adjuvant chemotherapy are nearing completion (ALPI, GETC, BLT etc.). Two small and methodologically less than ideal trials of neoadjuvant chemotherapy in stage III NSCLC (Rosell *et al.* 1994; Roth *et al.* 1994) have stimulated interest in this theoretically attractive approach and need to be confirmed in larger trials, for example LU22.

New drugs and drug combinations provide a further opportunity for advance and are being evaluated in large intergroup trials.

Adjuvant TI in completely resected patients with N0/N1 NSCLC is not beneficial and should not be used (PORT Meta-analysis Trialists Group 1998). Its role as an adjunct to surgery in patients with more advanced stages of tumour – N2 – is unclear and probably limited to improvements in local control, rather than having an impact on survival.

Combined modality therapy needs close collaboration between all the professional groups involved. Current plans for widespread implementation of multidisciplinary management of patients with lung cancer have a potential for making a real difference in this difficult disease with the largest survival gain coming from adoption of combined modality approach in appropriately selected groups of patients.

References

Aisner J, Forastierre A, Aroney R (1983). Patterns of recurrence for cancer of the lung and oesophagus. *Cancer Treatment Symposia* **2**, 87–105

American Society of Clinical Oncology (1997). Clinical practice guidelines for the treatment of unresectable non-small cell lung cancer. *Journal of Clinical Oncology* **15**, 1996–3018

Auperin A, Arriagada R, Pignon JP *et al.* (1999). Prophylactic cranial irradiation for patients with small cell lung cancer in complete remission: a meta-analysis of individual data from 987 patients. *New England Journal of Medicine* **341**, 476–484

Fergusson RJ, Gregor A, Dodds R, Kerr G (1996). Management of lung cancer in South East Scotland. *Thorax* **51**, 569–574

Ihde DC (1992). Chemotherapy of lung cancer. *New England Journal of Medicine* **327**, 1434–1441

Janssen-Heijnen MLG, Gatta G, Forman D *et al.* (1998). Variations in survival of patients with lung cancer in Europe, 1985-1989. *European Journal of Cancer* **34**, 2191–2196

Non-Small Cell Lung Cancer Collaborative Group (1995). Chemotherapy in non-small cell lung cancer; a meta- analysis using updated data on individual patients from 52 randomised trials. *British Medical Journal* **311**, 899–90

Pignon JP, Arriagada R, Ihde DC *et al.* (1992). A meta- analysis of thoracic radiotherapy for small cell lung cancer. *New England Journal of Medicine* **327**, 1618–1624

PORT Meta-analysis Trialists Group (1998). Postoperative radiotherapy in non-small-cell lung cancer: systematic review and meta-analysis of individual patient data from nine randomized controlled trials. *Lancet* **352**, 257–263

Rosell R, Gomez-Codina J, Camps C *et al.* (1994). A randomised trial comparing preoperative chemotherapy and surgery with surgery alone in patients with non-small cell lung cancer. *New England Journal of Medicine* **330**, 153–158

Roth JA, Fossella F, Komaki R *et al.* (1994). A randomised trial comparing perioperative chemotherapy and surgery with surgery alone in resectable stage III non small cell lung cancer. *Journal of the National Cancer Institute* **86**, 673–680

PART 3

Developing the evidence base: ongoing clinical trials

Chapter 8

Ongoing clinical trials for lung cancer in Europe and North America

Jeremy PC Steele and Robin M Rudd

Introduction

Cure rates for lung cancer remain low. For non-small cell lung cancer patients, cures can be achieved with radical surgery or radiotherapy or combinations of both; chemotherapy has not yet contributed significantly to the number of patients surviving. Chemotherapy can produce remissions in the majority of patients with small cell lung cancer but in the longterm only a small percentage are cured. In recent years, new drugs and new ways of delivering radiotherapy have led to fresh optimism in the search for better treatment results. Only well-organised clinical trials can establish the role of these new therapies.

Clinical trials in lung cancer have several possible endpoints: overall survival, progression-free survival, response rate and quality of life. In most phase III trials – including the majority of those discussed here – all four endpoints are examined. Quality of life has become a more commonly used endpoint and it is our view that all trials should include evaluation of quality of life.

Most trials are performed according to standard phase II and III designs. In the UK, trials take place within single institutions or on a multi-centre basis organised by collaborative groups such as the London Lung Cancer Group funded by the Cancer Research Campaign (CRC), and the Medical Research Council (MRC). Likewise, in mainland Europe, trials are conducted locally, nationally and internationally under the direction of groups such as the European Organization for Research and Treatment of Cancer (EORTC). In North America, the US and Canadian National Cancer Institutes co-ordinate and fund much trial activity. Other well-known collaborative groups in the US are the Southwest Oncology Group (SWOG), the Eastern Collaborative Oncology Group (ECOG) and the Cancer and Leukemia Group B (CALGB). Multi-centre trials have the advantage of centralised randomisation and data analysis and have the ability to recruit the large numbers of patients required for phase III studies.

This chapter describes some of the significant trials currently recruiting lung cancer patients in Europe and North America. No attempt has been made to be exhaustive and the trials discussed are included because they are attempting to answer important questions. In each case the trial is put in the context of the existing evidence base and the specific question being asked is highlighted. Possible difficulties with accrual, where present, are discussed. Trials in non-small cell lung cancer (NSCLC) are described first, followed by small cell lung cancer (SCLC).

Trials in non-small cell lung cancer

The accepted treatment approach for the medically fit patient with early-stage NSCLC (stages I and II) is radical surgery by lobectomy or pneumonectomy. Alternatively, radical thoracic radiotherapy can produce longterm cures in patients unsuitable for surgery. stage IIIA NSCLC is theoretically resectable but most patients are not cured. For patients with inoperable disease (i.e., stages IIIB and IV) treatment is palliative, although a recent meta-analysis showed a small survival benefit for patients treated with chemotherapy (Non-small Cell Lung Cancer Collaborative Group 1995). Thus there is an ongoing need to evaluate new ways of treating patients with this common type of cancer. Clinical trials designed to answer specific questions are an important method for improving outcomes for cancer patients. The key questions to be answered and some of the important trials addressing them are described below.

What is the role of pre-operative chemotherapy for patients with resectable (i.e., stages I-IIIA) non-small cell lung cancer?

Non-small cell lung cancer can be responsive to chemotherapy. Thus pre-operative chemotherapy would seem to be an attractive approach because it might shrink the tumour and make the subsequent surgery easier. Theoretically, there might also be a survival benefit due to elimination of undetectable metastases present at the time of diagnosis. Roth *et al.* (1994) reported a benefit for pre-operative chemotherapy, although the survival in the control arm (i.e., surgery only) appeared to be inferior to normal expectations. Rosell *et al.* (1994) described a similar result for patients treated with pre-operative chemotherapy, although there was an excess of poor-prognosis features in the control arm patient. Most collaborative groups feel that further trials are warranted. Trials attempting to answer this question include:

(1) Medical Research Council (MRC) Trial LU22 (UK)

Patients with resectable NSCLC are randomised to immediate surgery or to three cycles of pre-operative chemotherapy with either mitomycin, vinblastine, cisplatin (MVP), mitomycin, ifosfamide, cisplatin (MIC) or vinorelbine and cisplatin (NP). Accrual is currently 60 patients with a target of 450 and is below expectations.

(2) SWOG-9900 Trial (USA)

Patients with stages IB, II and selected IIIA NSCLC are randomised to immediate surgery or paclitaxel and carboplatin chemotherapy for up to three cycles and, pending toxicity, followed by surgery. Target accrual is 600 patients.

What is the role of post-operative chemotherapy and post-operative radiotherapy for patients with resected non-small cell lung cancer?

Adjuvant chemotherapy is known to be effective in breast and colon cancer but its value in NSCLC is not clear. The theoretical advantages are better longterm survival rates due to elimination of micrometastases as well as improved local control. Post-operative radiotherapy may also be beneficial, but data have been conflicting: indeed a recent meta-analysis suggested that radiotherapy might be detrimental (PORT Meta-analysis Trialists Group 1998). Trials attempting to answer these questions include:

(1) Adjuvant Lung Project (ALPI, Italy)

Patients with resected stages I–IIIA NSCLC were randomised to chemotherapy (three cycles of MVP: mitomycin $8mg/m^2$, vinblastine $3mg/m^2$ on days one and eight, cisplatin 100 mg/m^2) or no chemotherapy. Radiotherapy was given in either arm according to physician's discretion. This trial closed recently with 1,540 patients recruited and is under analysis.

(2) International Adjuvant Lung Trial (IALT, Europe)

Patients with operable (stages I-IIIA) NSCLC are randomised to chemotherapy or no chemotherapy after complete resection. Chemotherapy consists of cisplatin 80-$120mg/m^2$ plus one additional drug, either vinblastine, vindesine, vinorelbine or etoposide. Radiotherapy can be given to patients on either trial arm according to institutional guidelines. By September 1999, 1,578 of a planned 3,300 patients had been recruited with accrual anticipated to be complete by 2003.

(3) ANITA Studies 1 and 2 (Europe)

Patients with operable (stages I–IIIA) NSCLC after complete resection are randomised to chemotherapy or no chemotherapy. In ANITA 1, chemotherapy consists of vinorelbine $30mg/m^2$ and cisplatin $100mg/m^2$ and in ANITA 2, chemotherapy is single-agent vinorelbine. Radiotherapy is optional for patients with N2 disease. Accrual of ANITA 1 is almost complete at the time of writing.

(4) Phase III study of adjuvant chemotherapy for completely resected NSCLC NCIC/SWOG/ECOG/CALGB (North America)

Patients with resected T2 N0 or T1-2, N1 NSCLC are randomised to chemotherapy (vinorelbine $25mg/m^2$ weekly for 16 weeks plus cisplatin $50mg/m^2$ on days one and eight every four weeks for four cycles) or no further treatment. Target accrual is 600 patients over five years.

(5) Phase III study of chemotherapy with or without radiotherapy in patients with resected stage IIIA NSCLC (CALGB 9734, USA)

Patients with stage IIIA NSCLC (with N2 nodes only detected at operation) following complete resection are treated with four cycles of paclitaxel and carboplatin chemotherapy and then randomised to thoracic radiotherapy or no further treatment. Target accrual is 480 patients.

What is the best treatment policy for unresectable stage IIIA NSCLC?

Patients with inoperable stage IIIA NSCLC are traditionally offered radical thoracic radiotherapy with curative intent, although longterm survivors are few. There is therefore interest in adding chemotherapy to try and improve overall survival rates. There is also the chance that some patients will have a good response to chemotherapy and be rendered operable. The Medical Research Council (UK) attempted to answer these questions:

Unresectable stage IIIA NSCLC: a comparison of standard radiotherapy with chemotherapy followed by surgery or radiotherapy (MRC-LU20, UK)

Patients with untreated, unresectable stage IIIA NSCLC were randomised to receive standard thoracic radiotherapy or three drug combination chemotherapy (MVP or MIC according to investigator's preference) followed by radiotherapy or, if feasible, surgery. The target accrual was 350 patients over three years but the trial closed recently due to poor recruitment with only 48 patients randomised.

As with many trials in which the treatments in the two arms are substantially different, this trial closed due to slow accrual. It is also worth noting that patients with unresectable stage IIIA disease are a relatively small proportion of NSCLC in the UK where most patients present with clearly unresectable stage IIIB or IV disease.

Is surgery or radiotherapy better as definitive treatment for patients with stage IIIA NSCLC responding to initial chemotherapy?

For patients with operable stage IIIA NSCLC, surgery may offer a greater chance of longterm cure than radical radiotherapy (Ginsberg *et al.* 1997), although this question has not been systematically evaluated. Retrospective data suggest marginally superior survival rates for patients receiving surgery but this effect may be due to patient selection. Chemotherapy may also be beneficial to patients treated with stage IIIA disease prior to surgery or radiotherapy and the EORTC are addressing this issue in a randomised trial. This trial may suffer the accrual problems seen with the Medical Research Council study.

Chemotherapy followed by radiotherapy or surgery in stage IIIA (N2) NSCLC (EORTC-08941, Europe)

Patients with stage IIIA NSCLC receive three courses of any cisplatin or carboplatin-containing chemotherapy protocol. Patients achieving complete or partial remission are randomised to surgery or radiotherapy (60–62.5 Gy). In surgical patients, if resection margins or nodes are positive for tumour, post-operative radiotherapy will be given. The target accrual is 800 patients in order to randomise 400 patients.

What is the benefit of combining chemotherapy with continuous hyperfractionated accelerated radiotherapy (CHART) for patients with stage III NSCLC?

Continuous hyperfractionated accelerated radiotherapy (CHART) is radiotherapy given more than once daily such that the duration of treatment is shortened. Research protocols have examined twice or three times daily schedules of fractionation. Hyperfractionation has theoretical advantages in terms of improved tumour control derived from radiobiological models of tumour cell repopulation. The additional advantage for the patient is that the treatment period is halved (e.g., from five–six weeks of radiotherapy fractions to two–three weeks). Logistically, CHART places demands on radiotherapy departments because in order to achieve twice-daily fractions patients have to receive their first daily fraction early in the day in order that the second treatment be given at least six hours later (to maximise the radiobiological effect). Also, patients are required to remain in the vicinity of the hospital for the whole day rather than simply attend once.

Despite the significant financial and organisational issues there is considerable interest in CHART in Europe and North America because the original Mount Vernon trial of CHART in NSCLC showed improved overall survival and local control with acceptable toxicity (Saunders *et al.* 1997). Two ongoing trials are described:

(1) Chemotherapy followed by standard or hyperfractionated radiotherapy for unresectable stage IIIA or IIIB NSCLC (ECOG-2597, USA)

Patients with unresectable stage IIIA or IIIB NSCLC are treated with two cycles of paclitaxel and carboplatin chemotherapy. Responding patients and those with stable disease are randomised to standard or hyperfractionated (three fractions daily) radiotherapy (target accrual is 294 patients over three years).

(2) Phase II trial of hyperfractionated radiotherapy after chemotherapy (Mount Vernon, UK)

Patients with inoperable stage IIIA/IIIB NSCLC receive four cycles of cisplatin and paclitaxel followed by CHART.

What is the overall role of cisplatin-based chemotherapy in NSCLC and what are the quality of life benefits?

One trial is exploring the role of cisplatin-based chemotherapy at all stages of NSCLC: the London-based 'Big Lung Trial'. This large project allows the oncologist to randomise between the addition of chemotherapy and no further therapy for any patient with NSCLC for whom the value of chemotherapy is perceived to be uncertain or marginal.

Trial of cisplatin-based chemotherapy in NSCLC ('Big Lung Trial', London Lung Cancer Group, Europe)

A randomised trial to determine the value of cisplatin-based chemotherapy in NSCLC of any stage. Patients can have received surgery or radiotherapy or both or have advanced disease unsuitable for radical local therapy. In all settings the randomisation is between chemotherapy and no chemotherapy. Chemotherapy can be MIC, MVP, NP or cisplatin/vindesine (CV). Major endpoints are survival, progression-free survival, quality of life and health economics. Target accrual is 1,800 patients, 500 in the surgery group, 500 in the radical radiotherapy group and 800 in the supportive care group. As of September 2000, accrual stands at 306 in the surgery group, 241 in the radical radiotherapy group and 641 in the supportive care group.

Are newer chemotherapy drugs better or less toxic than existing agents?

Several new chemotherapy drugs have emerged in the last few years, some of which have shown useful activity in common solid tumours in adults. The most important of these are paclitaxel, gemcitabine, irinotecan and vinorelbine. Most newer agents have the additional advantage of being less toxic than older drugs. The most significant drawback is that all newer agents are several times the cost of the drugs they stand to supercede. Trials are ongoing aiming to determine the exact role of these newer drugs. Some examples are described below.

(1) Phase III trial of vinorelbine, gemcitabine or both in elderly patients with stage IIIB or stage IV NSCLC (EU-98019, Italy)

Elderly patients (defined as aged 70 years or older) with reasonable performance status are randomised to vinorelbine, gemcitabine or both on days one and eight of a three-week cycle. Patients not progressing after three cycles complete an additional three cycles. Endpoints are survival and quality of life. Target accrual is 630 patients.

(2) Phase III study of paclitaxel/cisplatin, gemcitabine/cisplatin or paclitaxel/gemcitabine in patients with advanced NSCLC (EORTC-08975, Europe)

Patients with advanced NSCLC, who may have had previous adjuvant chemotherapy, are randomised between one of the three arms. Endpoints are survival, toxicity and quality of life.

(3) Phase III trial comparing gemcitabine and carboplatin with mitomycin, ifosfamide and cisplatin in stage IIIB or IV NSCLC (London Lung Cancer Group Study 11, UK)

Patients receive chemotherapy with GC (gemcitabine 1200mg/m^2 on days one and eight and carboplatin AUC 5 on day one of a 21-day cycle) or MIC (mitomycin 6mg/m^2, ifosfamide 3g/m^2, cisplatin 50mg/m^2 on day one of a 21-day cycle). Endpoints are quality of life and survival. Target accrual is 387 patients.

Trials in small cell lung cancer

The chemosensitivity of small cell lung cancer (SCLC) is well established and the majority of patients – regardless of initial disease bulk – can be expected to achieve a partial or complete remission. However, only a small percentage (approximately 5 per cent) of individuals are cured and relapse after a period of months to years is normal. Clinical trial activity is aimed at prolongation of the progression-free period and increase in the number of cured patients. The important questions that need to be answered are:

What is the role of higher intensity treatment in patients with limited disease (LD) SCLC?

There has been interest in dose-intensified treatment for patients with SCLC for some years but results have not as yet been clear-cut (Elias 1998). Most investigators take the view that an optimally delivered platinum-containing protocol is the current gold standard and that higher dose or higher intensity therapy should only be used in clinical trials. Most current interest is centred on higher intensity chemotherapy rather than classical high dose therapy. Typically, growth factors are employed to allow chemotherapy cycles to be given two-weekly rather than the traditional three-weekly. Two examples of trials examining dose-intense therapy are described below.

(1) Phase II study of intensive chemotherapy with peripheral blood progenitor cell support (PBSC) in SCLC (EU-98072, Europe)

Patients with good prognosis SCLC are treated with four 14-day cycles of ifosfamide (day one) and carboplatin (day one) and etoposide (days one and two); G-CSF is administered subcutaneously from day two until blood cell counts recover. Peripheral blood progenitor cells are harvested after cycle one and reinfused after cycles two and three. Patients achieving complete remission will receive prophylactic cranial radiotherapy (an accrual of 36 patients is expected over 18 months).

(2) Phase III trial of VICE chemotherapy versus standard treatment in SCLC (MRC-LU21 trial, UK)

Patients with limited disease SCLC or good-prognosis extensive SCLC receive six courses of intensive VICE chemotherapy (ifosfamide $5g/m^2$, carboplatin $300mg/m^2$, etoposide $120mg/m^2$ on day one and vincristine $1mg/m^2$ on day 14, repeated every 28 days) or standard chemotherapy (either doxorubicin, cyclophosphamide, etoposide (ACE) or cisplatin and etoposide (PE)) for six courses. Target accrual is 400 patients of which 261 had been accrued by the end of 1999.

When should radiotherapy be administered in limited disease SCLC?

Data have suggested that thoracic radiotherapy for patients with limited disease SCLC is more beneficial if administered synchronously (Murray *et al.* 1993), although acute toxicity is greater. The trial described below should clarify the issue but has had problems with slow accrual:

Phase III trial to examine the optimum timing of thoracic radiotherapy in limited disease SCLC (London Lung Cancer Group Study 8, UK)

Patients with limited, good performance status small volume disease SCLC are all treated with CAV/PE (cyclophosphamide, doxorubicin and vincristine alternating with cisplatin and etoposide) chemotherapy and prophylactic cranial radiotherapy and are randomised between 40 Gy of thoracic radiotherapy given after the first cycle of PE or after the third cycle of PE. Of a target of 320 patients, 240 have been recruited.

What is the benefit of newer chemotherapy agents?

Newer agents such as paclitaxel, docetaxel, gemcitabine, irinotecan and vinorelbine have demonstrated activity in SCLC and are being tested in randomised trials. All of these agents appear to have useful single-agent activity in SCLC but are considerably more expensive than existing drugs.

(1) Phase III study of etoposide and cisplatin with or without paclitaxel in extensive disease SCLC (National Cancer Institute and CALGB-9732, USA)

Patients with extensive disease SCLC are randomised to six three-weekly cycles of PE or PE plus additional paclitaxel on day one with G-CSF on days 4–18. Target accrual is 670 patients over 16 months.

(2) Gemcitabine/carboplatin compared with cisplatin/etoposide in extensive disease and poor-prognosis limited disease SCLC patients (London Lung Cancer Group Study 10, UK)

Patients with SCLC (extensive disease or limited disease with poor-prognosis factors) are randomised to six cycles of gemcitabine 1200mg/m^2 on days one and eight and carboplatin AUC 5 on day one or six cycles of cisplatin 60mg/m^2 and etoposide 120mg/m^2 IV on day one and 100mg twice daily PO on days two and three). Endpoints are response, quality of life and survival. Target accrual is 241 patients.

Should second-line therapy for patients with SCLC be routine?

Second-line treatment of patients with SCLC is of uncertain value, although many oncologists feel that the symptomatic benefit for selected patients can be significant. One standard approach is to re-treat the patient with a platinum-based combination though some centres are investigating the role of newer, non-cross resistant agents in this setting.

(1) Phase II trial of an outpatient schedule of irinotecan, cisplatin and mitomycin C (IPM) in relapsed SCLC (St Bartholomew's Hospital, London)

Patients with recurrent SCLC are treated with irinotecan 70mg/m^2 and cisplatin 40mg/m^2, two-weekly and mitomycin C 6mg/m^2 four-weekly for up to six cycles according to response. Initial accrual will be 24 patients.

(2) Phase II trial of topotecan and paclitaxel in relapsed SCLC (National Cancer Institute, USA)

Patients with recurrent SCLC are treated with paclitaxel and topotecan in cohorts with escalating doses of topotecan for a maximum of six courses.

Are new treatment modalities of value?

Because standard cytotoxic treatments have such low cure rates, SCLC is an ideal disease in which to assess treatments of a more experimental nature. Novel approaches such as anti-angiogenesis, monoclonal antibody targeting and gene therapy are being evaluated in SCLC. All of these strategies remain investigational and should not be used outside the setting of a clinical trial. In some countries gene therapy protocols are monitored by government agencies. Some examples are given below:

(1) Marimastat following response to chemotherapy in SCLC (EORTC and National Cancer Institute of Canada, Europe and North America)

Patients with limited disease SCLC who had responded to chemotherapy and then received thoracic radiotherapy and prophylactic cranial irradiation were randomised to marimastat (a matrix metalloproteinase inhibitor) 10 mg twice daily or placebo for two years or until progression. The study closed at the end of 1999 with 540 patients recruited and is under analysis.

(2) SILVA study in SCLC (EORTC Lung Cancer Group Trial 08971, Europe)

Patients with limited disease SCLC who have responded to chemotherapy and then received thoracic radiotherapy and prophylactic cranial irradiation are randomised to observation or to five intradermal vaccinations over ten weeks of BCG plus BEC2, an anti-idiotype monoclonal antibody which induces antibodies to GD3, a ganglioside present in SCLC. The end-point is survival and 570 patients are required. The study has just started recruiting.

(3) Phase II trial of carboplatin/etoposide and thalidomide in SCLC (London Lung Cancer Group, UK)

Patients are treated with six cycles of carboplatin and etoposide with thalidomide 100 mg orally daily for up to two years. Thoracic radiotherapy and prophylactic cranial irradiation may be used as appropriate. Endpoints are response, toxicity, progression-free survival, overall survival and quality of life. Drug-induced DNA damage and anti-angiogenesis parameters are also being evaluated. Initial accrual will be 24 patients.

(4) Phase II pilot study of tumour-specific p53 or ras vaccines with or without cellular immunotherapy with peptide-activated lymphocytes plus interleukin-2 (NCI, USA)

Patients with lung, pancreatic, breast, colon, cervical and ovarian cancer can be entered into this trial. All patients are required to have a detectable p53 or ras mutation, insertion or deletion. Patients are vaccinated with antigen-presenting cells pulsed in vitro with synthetic peptide corresponding to the tumour's p53 or ras mutation to assess if the patient's cellular immunity can be boosted. The ability of primed T cells (generated by this vaccination with interleukin-2 enhancement) to enhance cytotoxic T lymphocyte immune response in vivo will be evaluated.

Can cytoprotective agents and cytokines reduce the toxicity of chemotherapy?

Although there are promising new approaches to lung cancer therapy under evaluation, chemotherapy remains the mainstay of drug treatment for the foreseeable future. Agents that have the ability to attenuate the toxicities of chemotherapy are being tested in pilot studies and phase II trials.

(1) Amifostine in NSCLC and SCLC (USA and UK)

This compound is known to reduce some of the toxicities of cisplatin and some alkylating agents. It is being tested in combination with various cytotoxics and in several tumour types.

(2) Erythropoietin to prevent anaemia in patients on chemotherapy for lung cancer (multi-centre European trial)

Erythropoietin is of proven value in the maintenance of red blood cell counts in patients with chronic renal failure and therefore is a logical drug to assess in patients having chemotherapy for lung cancer in whom anaemia is a source of significant morbidity. Multicentre international trials are in progress.

Conclusions

There are large numbers of clinical trials in lung cancer in progress in North America and Europe. If recruitment to trials continues, it is possible that many of the important questions regarding the best management of NSCLC and SCLC with surgery, chemotherapy and radiotherapy will be answered in the next few years. New modalities of therapy offer promise but most are at an early stage of development. It is our view that clinical trials should receive maximal support from governments, healthcare systems and physicians. As many patients as possible should have the opportunity to be treated within a clinical trial.

*References*_____

Elias A (1998). Dose-intensive therapy in small cell lung cancer. *Chest* **113**, 101S–106S

Ginsberg RJ, Vokes EE, Raben A (1997). Non-small cell lung cancer. *In Cancer, Principles and Practice of Oncology, Fifth Edition.* DeVita VT, Hellman S, Rosenberg SA (eds) Philadelphia and New York: Lippincott-Raven, pp. 858–911

Murray N, Coy P, Pater JL *et al.* (1993). Importance of timing for thoracic irradiation in the combined modality treatment of limited-stage small-cell lung cancer. The National Cancer Institute of Canada Clinical Trials Group. *Journal of Clinical Oncology* **11**, 336–344

Non-small Cell Lung Cancer Collaborative Group (1995). Chemotherapy in non-small cell lung cancer: a meta-analysis using updated data on individual patients from 52 randomised clinical trials. *British Medical Journal* **311**, 899–909

PORT Meta-analysis Trialists Group. (1998). Postoperative radiotherapy in non-small-cell lung cancer: systematic review and meta-analysis of individual patient data from nine randomised trials. *Lancet* **352**, 257–263

Roth JA, Fossella F, Komaki R *et al.* (1994). A randomized trial comparing perioperative chemotherapy and surgery with surgery alone in resectable stage IIIA non-small-cell lung cancer. *Journal of the National Cancer Institute* **86**, 673–680

Rosell R, Gomez-Codina J, Camps C *et al.* (1994). A randomized trial comparing preoperative chemotherapy plus surgery with surgery alone in patients with non-small-cell lung cancer. *New England Journal of Medicine* **330**, 153–158

Saunders M, Dische S, Barrett A *et al.* (1997). Continuous hyperfractionated accelerated radiotherapy (CHART) versus conventional radiotherapy in non-small-cell lung cancer: a randomised multicentre trial. *Lancet* **350**, 161–165

PART 4

Current debate on dose intensification and the evidence base for palliative intervention

Chapter 9

Dose intensification of chemotherapy in small cell lung cancer: the case for

Sacha J Howell, Rhada Bhaskaran, Mark R Middleton and
Nicholas Thatcher

Introduction

The clinical value of dose intensification in SCLC has recently been the subject of a number of randomised controlled trials. Pre-clinical models, particularly the work of Skipper *et al.* (1970) and Schabel *et al.* (1984), established the relationship between dose factors and tumour response. The work indicated that the dose response curve for the majority of anti-tumour agents was usually steep in the linear phase. Importantly, it was determined from these data that a dose reduction of approximately 20 per cent could lead to a reduction of cure of 50 per cent or more. In contrast, a two-fold increase in the dose could lead to a ten-fold increase in tumour cell kill (De Vita 1989, 1991; Gurney *et al.* 1993a). Skipper (1990) also reported a retrospective analysis of the original data , which indicated that dose intensity affects the degree of response achieved, whereas cumulative dose correlates more with survival time. It can be inferred therefore that increased dose intensity for a short period is desirable when cure is intended but lower dose intensity for a longer period is preferable for palliation.

The older clinical reports, which in general showed no relationship between total dose, dose intensity and survival, were analysed on planned protocol doses rather than the actual dose received by the patient. As many of the 'high dose intensity' regimens had doses reduced due to patient toxicity, the received dose intensity in these trials was almost always less than that in the standard arm. Therefore, in many of these studies the relationship between dose intensity and survival was not adequately assessed. Nevertheless SCLC is a very chemosensitive tumour and somatic models predict the probability of developing drug resistance with time (Coldman & Goldie 1987; De Vita 1991). These models suggest that the probability of developing drug resistance due to random mutations in later dosing is greatly reduced by higher initial doses of chemotherapy. In addition, dose intensive regimens should reduce tumour growth between treatments, allowing fewer mutants to arise during chemotherapy, and meaning longterm remissions or cures should be more frequent. It is a logical conclusion, therefore, to treat with maximal chemotherapy doses in the first instance with the shortest possible intervals between treatments.

Retrospective analyses of dose intensity

There have been a number of retrospective analyses concerning the relationship between dose intensity (defined as mgs/m^2 per week) and outcome. The meta-analysis by Klasa et al. (1991) examined sixty published studies. Increased dose intensity in the cyclophosphamide, doxorubicin, vincristine, etoposide (CAVE) and cyclophosphamide, doxorubicin, etoposide (CAE) regimens correlated positively with median survival in extensive stage disease. This was not so with the cyclophosphamide, doxorubicin, vincristine (CAV) regimen nor with other comparisons. Another study of extensive stage patients who received CAV-type regimens at conventional doses or at a higher dose intensity reported significantly better one year survival rates (32 per cent versus 12 per cent) and overall survival with the higher dose intensity (Sheehan et al. 1993). A recent analysis of two consecutive phase II studies in 131 limited stage patients has been reported. The two studies used the same four drugs (etoposide, cyclophosphamide, doxorubicin, cisplatin) in an alternating radiotherapy/chemotherapy schedule. In the multivariate analysis the five-year survival rate was 25 per cent if higher initial doses of cisplatin and cyclophosphamide were given but only 9 per cent (p<0.01) for the other patients treated with lower doses (De Vathaire et al. 1993).

If toxicity requires dose modification it may be better to maintain the dose but increase the interval between chemotherapy courses, rather than reduce the dose, which is common practice (Gurney et al. 1993b). The Manchester group has examined the combination of ifosfamide, carboplatin and etoposide with mid-course vincristine (VICE) in three consecutive phase II studies totalling 166 patients. Inclusion criteria required a reasonable performance status but both limited and extensive stage disease were accepted (Thatcher et al. 1989; Prendiville et al. 1991, 1994). An important policy was that no dose reduction over a total of six chemotherapy courses was adopted. This strategy has produced survival rates of over 30 per cent with a minimum follow up of at least two years. Further analysis has demonstrated a five-year survival rate of 19 per cent with a minimum follow up of four and a half years (Thatcher et al. 1994; Lorigan et al. 1995). Dose intensity was maintained with the policy of dose delay rather than dose reduction. Despite the myelotoxicity most of the patients received all six courses of chemotherapy at full dose. However, when cisplatin was alternated with carboplatin, fewer courses were given, a lower percentage of patients received all six courses and there was increased toxicity mainly due to renal impairment (Prendiville et al. 1991). Table 9.1 shows that the protocol dose intensity can be maintained with this policy both over the first three and also subsequent cycles. If both dose delay and dose reduction are practised the relative dose intensity is reduced, as shown in the London study (Smith et al. 1990). Again, when only four courses of chemotherapy were given together with dose reduction a poorer two-year survival rate was obtained even though a similar population of patients were treated (Hatton et al. 1995). Despite the bone marrow toxicity of the VICE regimen the patients' performance status and disease related symptoms improved rapidly (Thatcher et al. 1989, 1994; Prendiville et al. 1991, 1994;

Table 9.1 Relative dose intensity with VICE-type chemotherapy

Reference	Regimen	RDI courses 1–3	RDI courses 4–6	Patients given 6 cycles (%)	Median survival (months)	2-year survival (%)
Thatcher et al. (1989)	VICE	1	1	74	14	33
Prendiville (1991)	VIC/PE†	1	0.77	68	14	30
Prendiville et al. (1994)	VICE†	1	0.86	72	16	31
Smith et al. (1990)	ICE‡	0.92	0.66	72	13	22
Hatton et al. (1995)	ICE‡	Only four courses given			10	11

† Intercalated Radiotherapy
‡ Dose Reduction Practised
Key: V=vincristine, I=ifosfamide, C=carboplatin, E=etoposide, p=cisplatin
RDI=Relative Dose Intensity

Lorrigan et al. 1995). These parameters of therapeutic efficacy are rarely reported with intensive regimens and should be considered alongside the conventional grading of haematological and other toxicities, which are usually transient.

Prospective randomised trials

As previously stated, early studies of increased dose intensity were flawed, either due to analyses based on proposed rather than achieved dose intensity or to underdosing by today's standards in the 'standard intensity' arms. These earlier studies arose from the trial of Cohen et al. (1977), which reported significantly improved response rate and survival when the dose of cyclophosphamide was increased from 0.5–1 gram /m^2; lomustine from 50–100 mgs/m^2 and methotrexate from 10–15 mgs/m^2. However, the chemotherapy doses in the standard arm of this trial would now be considered suboptimal. More recently, a prospective French trial of a four drug regimen, based on an earlier retrospective study (De Vathaire et al. 1993), randomised patients to receive cisplatin and cyclophosphamide at increased dose (by 33 per cent and 20 per cent respectively) for the first of six courses of chemotherapy only. The doses of doxorubicin and etoposide were identical for both groups. The first course of chemotherapy was followed by five additional standard dose courses with three inter-collated courses of radiotherapy. At two years, survival was increased from 26–43 per cent (p=0.008 on multivariate analysis) for the patients receiving the higher dose chemotherapy (Arriagada et al. 1993).

As the growth fraction of a tumour may increase with tumour response to treatment, the intensity of therapy that results in regression may be insufficient to sustain that response. Norton and Simon (1977) therefore suggest that chemotherapy should be intensified as soon as possible for as long as possible after standard induction treatment. The success of late intensification in haematological malignancies with bone marrow transplantation encouraged the use of a similar approach in chemoresponsive tumours such as SCLC. Following tumour remission with conventional treatment high dose chemotherapy was administered which required hospitalisation and full supportive care. Studies of this technique have used very limited patient numbers and, although complete responses have been increased, no obvious survival improvement has been noted. In a review of 178 patients from seven studies, 37 per cent had a complete response after the late intensification procedure but only 9.5 per cent of patients were alive one year after therapy and 7.8 per cent died during treatment (Klastersky & Sculier 1989).

Humblet *et al.* (1987) performed the only randomised study of high-dose against conventional-dose chemotherapy, all patients having responded to induction with conventional dose regimes. The high-dose regime of cyclophosphamide ($6gm/m^2$), etoposide ($500mg/m^2$) and carmustine ($300mg/m^2$) followed by autologous bone marrow transplantation, increased relapse-free survival from 10 to 28 weeks although the increase in overall survival from 55 to 68 weeks did not achieve statistical significance. There are inherent problems in randomised trials of late intensification in that very large numbers of patients are required. Only about one third of patients in late intensification programmes are suitable for the procedure because of toxicity during the induction regimen, lack of initial response or inability to withstand the side-effects of late intensification chemotherapy. The development of recombinant haemopoietic growth factors has allowed intensive accelerated chemotherapy to be given without the need for bone marrow transplantation.

Dose intensification with G-CSF and GM-CSF

Myelosuppression is the commonest dose-limiting toxicity previously preventing exploration of increased dose intensity. There is now ample evidence that haemopoietic growth factors can be used for dose intensification. Trillet-Lenoir *et al.* (1993) showed that G-CSF reduced the need for dose reduction with cyclophosphamide, doxorubicin, etoposide (CDE). Dose reductions were needed in 61 per cent of controls, but only 29 per cent of those on G-CSF ($p<0.001$). When doses are delayed, rather than reduced for toxicity, G-CSF allows intensification of this drug combination. Over four hundred patients were randomised to receive chemotherapy every three weeks or every two weeks with G-CSF in a trial run by the British Medical Research Council. Dose intensity was increased by 33 per cent with G-CSF; these patients completed treatment sooner than, and with similar toxicity to, the control arm. One- and two-year survival were also significantly improved in the G-CSF arm (47

Table 9.2 Randomised phase III trials of accelerated chemotherapy with and without G-CSF and GM-CSF

Ref.	Regimen	stage + Pt.No. LS	ES	CR(%)	PR(%)	MS (months)	2 year survival	RDI (%)
Miles *et al.* (1994)	PE/IA vs.	12	5	71%OR		NR	NR	82
	PE/IA + G-CSF	15	8	74%OR		NR	NR	84
Fukuoka *et al.* (1997) †	CODE vs. CODE +	–	31	23	61	8.0	6.5%	72
	G-CSF	–	32	34	63	14.8	31%	84
Woll *et al.* (1995)	VICE vs.	28	3	58	36	16.3	15%	118
	VICE + G-CSF	32	2	56	38	17.3	32%	125
Furuse *et al.* (1998)	CAV/PE vs.	–	113	15	61	10.9	8.5%	82
	CODE + G-CSF	–	114	16	68	11.6	11.7%	72
Steward *et al.* (1998) † ‡	VICE q4w vs.	85	68	41	24	12.5	18%	NR
	VICE q3w	93	54	44	33	15.8	33%	126
Thatcher *et al.* (2000) †	ACE q3w vs. ACE q2w	151	51	28	50	11.8	8%	NR
	+ G-CSF	153	48	40	38	12.5	13%	134%

† statistically significant survival advantage

‡ second randomisation to receive GM-CSF or not

CODE cisplatin /vincristine /doxorubicin /etoposide

CAV cyclophosphamide /doxorubicin /vincristine

VICE vincristine /ifosfamide /carboplatin /etoposide

ACE doxorubicin /cyclophosphamide /etoposide

PE cisplatin /etoposide

IA ifosfamide /doxorubicin

G-CSF granulocyte colony stimulating factor

GM-CSF granulocyte macrophage colony stimulating factor

CR complete response, PR partial response, OR overall response

LS limited stage, ES extensive stage, MS median survival, NR not reported

RDI relative dose intensity

Table 9.3 Trials of weekly chemotherapy

phase II Studies

Ref.	Regimen	Pt.No	stage	CR(%)	PR(%)	MS (months)
Taylor *et al.*	CD/MV/P	34	LS	47	35	16.6
(1990)	E/V	42	ES	38	43	11.4
Miles *et al.*	PE/IA	45	LS	51	40	14.5
(1991)		25	ES	48	44	10.5
Murray *et al.*	CODE	48	ES	40	54	15.2
(1991)						

Randomised phase III Studies

Ref	Regimen	Pt.No	stage	CR(%)	PR(%)	MS (months)	2-year survival	RDI
Sculier	ACE q3w	48	LS	21	37	10.8	8.5%	
et al.	vs.	60	ES					
(1993)	ACE/Vd							-14%
	P/VM	47	LS	31	41	12.3	7.9%	
	weekly	60	ES					
Souhami	CAV/PE	135	LS	39	43	10.6	11.7%	
et al.	q3w vs.	82	ES					
(1994)								-20%
	IA/PE	141	LS	37	44	10.8	11.8%	
	weekly	80	ES					
Murray *et al.*	CAV/PE	109	ES	22	47	11.9	18%	
1999	q3w vs.							200%
	CODE	110	ES	27	60	12.8	18%	
	weekly							

C = cyclophosphamide unless part of CODE when C = cisplatin
D or A=doxorubicin, M=methotrexate, V or O=vincristine, p=cisplatin, E=etoposide
I=ifosfamide, Vd=vindesine, LS=limited stage, ES=extensive stage, CR=complete response,
PR=partial respnse, MS=median Survival, RDI=relative dose intensity

per cent versus 37 per cent and 13 per cent versus 8 per cent respectively; $p=0.04$ (Thatcher *et al.* 2000) (Table 9.2).

The choice of chemotherapeutic agents and their schedule of administration appear to be of great importance with regard to the ability to achieve the proposed increase in dose intensity and the translation of this increased dose intensity into an improvement in survival. Several attempts have been made to increase dose intensity using weekly chemotherapy schedules. The results of several of these are summarised in Table 9.3. In the study by Souhami *et al.* (1994), 48 patients were randomised to receive either weekly chemotherapy of ifosfamide/doxorubicin alternating with cisplatin/etoposide, or cyclophosphamide, adriamycin, vincristine (CAV) and cisplatin, etoposide (PE) alternating on a three-weekly basis. There were no significant differences in response rates or survival between the treatment groups, for extensive or limited stage disease. Dose intensity was only slightly increased in the weekly treatment arm, further increase prevented by haematological toxicity. The addition of G-CSF to this regime, in a phase II study by the same investigators (Miles *et al.* 1994), typifies the low success rates of dose intensification with cisplatin containing combinations. They randomised 40 good prognosis ES and LS-SCLC patients to receive G-CSF or not during treatment with weekly alternating cisplatin/etoposide and ifosfamide/doxorubicin. Received dose intensity was 84 per cent of that projected in the G-CSF arm and 82 per cent in the unsupported arm, despite a significant decrease in dose-reductions in the G-CSF arm. Renal toxicity was the predominant non-haematological toxicity preventing escalation of received dose intensity.

Substitution of cisplatin with carboplatin has several theoretical advantages. Most importantly, carboplatin has reduced renal and neuro-toxicity compared with cisplatin, thus, despite the relative increase in transient myelotoxicity, dose intensification is possible with blood product and growth factor support. The first paper on the VICE regime came from Manchester (Thatcher *et al.* 1989) in relatively poor prognosis patients of both limited and extensive stage. Median survival of the entire group was 14 months and actual two-year survival was 33 per cent. The large study of Steward *et al.* (1998) randomised patients to three or four weekly VICE, with or without GM-CSF (a second double-blind randomisation). Although the addition of GM-CSF did not significantly reduce the incidence of complications from myelosuppression, nor improve survival, the dose-intensification of VICE to three-weekly was superior to the four-weekly regime in terms of median survival (14.4 versus 11.5 months; $p=0.0014$) and two-year survival (33 per cent versus 18 per cent). A 26 per cent increase in dose intensity was achieved in the three-weekly regime compared with the four-weekly, and the addition of GM-CSF produced a trend for greater dose intensity. Importantly, as with all of the Manchester group's trials, doses were not reduced but weekly dose delay was employed to allow recovery from myelosuppression. This policy, discussed by Lorigan *et al.* (1995), results in less reduction in dose intensity compared with that of dose reduction and delay, with no significant increase in toxicity.

Several other attempts have been made to increase dose intensity with GCSF. Of particular note is the study by Woll *et al.*(1995) (Table 9.2), who randomised 65 patients to VICE with or without G-CSF. Dose intensity was increased above that of the standard four- weekly schedule in both arms by giving chemotherapy as soon as the blood counts had recovered adequately. No dose reductions were performed over the six cycles of planned therapy. The G-CSF group received a significantly higher dose intensity than the control group (no G-CSF) with greatest dose intensity difference in the first three cycles (134 per cent versus 117 per cent, $p=0.01$). For all six cycles the dose intensity was 125 per cent for G-CSF patients and 118 per cent for controls. The median survival of 65 weeks for the controls and 69 weeks for G-CSF patients was not significantly different, but the proportion of patients alive at two years was 32 per cent for the G-CSF higher dose intensity regimen compared with 15 per cent for the controls.

Dose intensification with peripheral blood progenitor cell support

Further dose escalation even with the ICE/VICE regimes is problematic because of thrombocytopenia. However, an important method of reducing myelotoxicity overall is to utilise peripheral blood progenitor cells (PBPC). They are mobilised from bone marrow in significant numbers during normal recovery from myelosuppressive chemotherapy and this process can be augmented by the administration of G and GM-CSF. Unlike the situation in lymphoma and other rare tumours, the requirement for technical expertise and equipment, needed for cell separation, cryopreservation and thawing, prevents the use of leucopheresis to support dose intensification therapy in common cancers. The Manchester Group have reported on the viability of harvested PBPC in both whole blood and leucopheresis product stored for 48 hours at 4°C. The viability of the cells was similar to that found after conventional cryopreservation and thawing. This suggested that PBPC in whole blood could be stored for limited periods at 4°C and used to support multicyclic chemotherapy (Pettengell *et al.* 1994).

These observations led to the initiation of a cohort study with three groups of patients in which haemopoietic progenitors were collected following chemotherapy and G-CSF stimulation, stored either by cryopreservation or at 4°C in a blood fridge and reinfused on day three of the subsequent chemotherapy cycle. The first cohort was treated every three weeks, with leukopheresis and cryopreservation every two weeks post-chemotherapy. The second cohort was treated every two weeks, with leukopheresis immediately prior to chemotherapy and storage of the product at 4°C until reinfusion. The third cohort was also treated every two weeks but with 500–750 mls of whole blood drawn by venesection immediately prior to chemotherapy and stored at 4°C prior to reinfusion. Each procedure was repeated for every cycle of chemotherapy.

Results showed that the myelosuppressive ICE regimen could be given every two weeks at full dose over six cycles using peripheral blood progenitor cell whole blood autotransfusions after each cycle. The technique achieved a 190–200 per cent dose intensification (Pettengell *et al.* 1995). Following this a randomised phase II study was performed in which 50 patients with SCLC with good prognosis were allocated to receive standard four-weekly ICE chemotherapy or two-weekly treatment with peripheral progenitor cell autotransfusion support. There was a substantial increase in relative dose intensity of 180 per cent in the autotransfusion arm compared with the standard regimen ($p=0.0001$). Surprisingly, toxicity and the requirement for antibiotics and hospitalisation was less for patients receiving the intensified treatment with autotransfusions (Woll *et al.* 1996). A randomised phase III study is currently in progress to test whether this novel dose intensification approach confers a survival benefit over standard treatment.

New growth factors and marrow protection

There are a number of haemopoietic growth factors in development. IL-3, IL-6 and IL-11 have all shown activity in the treatment of chemotherapy-induced thrombocytopaenia (Crawford & George 1995; Kudoh *et al.* 1996; Tepler *et al.* 1996]. Erythropoietin is reported to be effective in the treatment and prevention of anaemia associated with chemotherapy (Case *et al.* 1993; De Campos *et al.* 1995). However, to date no studies have examined the role of these drugs in intensifying treatment. Treatment with combinations of growth factors is feasible (Crawford & George 1995), despite overlapping toxicities, and the use of agents in development is likely to be in combination with existing approaches, rather than replacing them.

An alternative approach to intensifying myelosuppressive chemotherapy lies in inducing resistance in the marrow stem cell population to chemotherapy. This has been demonstrated in animals treated with chloroethylnitrosoureas, whose DNA-damaging effects are counteracted by the repair protein O^6-alkylguanine-DNA alkyltransferase (ATase). Toxicity due to carmustine was significantly reduced in mice whose bone marrow cells were removed, a bacterial ATase gene introduced, and then replaced prior to treatment (Harris *et al.* 1995). This approach will generalise to other resistance factors, with applicability to SCLC treatments. Myelosuppression might also be avoided by switching stem cells into a holding, rather than proliferative, mode at the time of chemotherapy. Since rapidly dividing cells are the target for many chemotherapeutic drugs this can attenuate haematological toxicity. This approach has been tested in murine models, using macrophage inflammatory protein-1α (MIP-1α), an inhibitor of primitive stem cells (Lord *et al.* 1992). Not all drugs, however, are specific for cells in the DNA synthesis phase but this approach merits further investigation as a means to intensify treatment.

Conclusions

One of the major issues for the development of dose-intense treatment of SCLC lies in the acceptability of such therapy to patients and health care purchasers. Patient acceptance of intensified treatment is good; indeed cancer sufferers are more accepting of potentially toxic treatments than their physicians and other health professionals (Slevin *et al.* 1990). However, quality of life analyses should be considered in studies of dose intensification strategies. Attainment of the increased levels of dose intensification now possible could bring the goal of increased longterm survival in SCLC closer.

References

Arriagada R, Le Chevalier T, Pignon J-P *et al.* (1993). Initial chemotherapeutic doses and survival in patients with limited small cell lung cancer. *New England Journal of Medicine* **329**, 1848–1852

Case DC, Bukowski RM, Carey RW *et al.* (1993). Recombinant human erythropoietin therapy for anaemic cancer patients on combination chemotherapy. *Journal of the National Cancer Institute* **85**, 801–806

Cohen MH, Creaven PJ, Fossieck BE (1977). Intensive chemotherapy of small cell bronchogenic carcinoma. *Cancer Treatment Reports* **61**, 349–354

Coldman AJ & Goldie JH (1987). Impact of dose-intense chemotherapy on the development of permanent drug resistance. *Seminars in Oncology* **14**, 29–33

Crawford J & George M (1995). The role of haematopoietic growth factors in support of ifosfamide/carboplatin/etoposide chemotherapy. *Seminars in Oncology* **22**, 18–22

De Campos E, Radford J, Steward W *et al.* (1995). Clinical and in vitro effects of recombinant human erythropoietin in patients receiving intensive chemotherapy for small-cell lung cancer. *Journal of Clinical Oncology* **13**, 1623–1631

De Vathaire F, Arriagada R, De The H *et al.* (1993). Dose intensity of initial chemotherapy may have an impact on survival in limited small cell lung carcinoma. *Lung Cancer* **8**, 301–308

DeVita VT (1989). Principles of chemotherapy in DeVita VT, Hellman S, Rosenberg SA (eds) *Cancer, Principles and Practice of Oncology*. Philadelphia: JB Lippincott. pp.276–300

DeVita VT (1991). The influence of information on drug resistance on protocol design. *Annals of Oncology* **2**, 93–106

Fukuoka M, Masuda N, Negoro S *et al.* (1997). CODE chemotherapy with and without granulocyte colony stimulating factor in small cell lung cancer. *British Journal of Cancer* **75**, 306–309

Furuse K, Fukuoka M, Nishiwaki Y *et al.* (1998). phase III study of intensive weekly chemotherapy with recombinant human granulocyte colony-stimulating factor versus standard chemotherapy in extensive-disease small-cell lung cancer. *Journal of Clinical Oncology* **16**, 2126–2132

Gurney H, Dodwell D, Thatcher N *et al.* (1993). Escalating drug delivery in cancer chemotherapy: A review of concepts and practice - part 1. *Annals of Oncology* **4**, 23–34

Gurney H, Dodwell D, Thatcher N *et al.* (1993). Escalating drug delivery in cancer chemotherapy: A review of concepts and practice - Part 2. *Annals of Oncology* **4**, 103–115

Harris LC, Marathi UK, Edwards CC *et al.* (1995). Retroviral transfer of a bacterial alkyltransferase gene into murine bone marrow protects against chloroethylnitrosourea cytotoxicity. *Clinical Cancer Research* **1**, 1359–1368

Hatton MQF, Cassidy J, Bicknell S *et al.* (1995). Ifosphamide, carboplatin and etoposide for good prognosis small cell lung cancer. Are four courses adequate? *European Journal of Cancer* **31A**, 1022–1023

Humblet Y, Symann M, Bosly A *et al.* (1987). Late intensification chemotherapy with autologous bone marrow transplantation in selected small-cell carcinoma of the lung: a randomized study. *Journal of Clinical Oncology* **5**, 1864–73

Klasa RJ, Murray N, Coldman AJ (1991). Dose intensity meta-analysis of chemotherapy regimens in small cell carcinoma of the lung. *Journal of Clinical Oncology* **9**, 499–508

Klastersky JA & Sculier JP (1989). Intensive chemotherapy of small cell lung cancer. *Lung Cancer* **5**, 196–206

Kudoh S, Sawa T, Kurihara N *et al.* (1996). phase II study of recombinant human interleukin 3 administration following carboplatin and etoposide chemotherapy in small-cell lung cancer patients. *Cancer Chemotherapy and Pharmacology* **38**, S89–S95

Lord BI, Dexter TM, Clements JM *et al.* (1992). Macrophage inflammatory protein protects multipotent haemopoietic cells from the cytotoxic effects of hydroxyurea in vivo. *Blood* **79**, 2605–2609

Lorigan P, Ming Lee S, Betticher D *et al.* (1995). Chemotherapy with vincristine / ifosphamide / carboplatin / etoposide in small cell lung cancer. *Seminars in Oncology* **22**, 32–41

Miles DW, Earl HM, Souhami RL *et al.* (1991). Intensive weekly chemotherapy for good-prognosis patients with small-cell lung cancer. *Journal of Clinical Oncology* **9**, 280–285

Miles DW, Fogarty O, Ash CM *et al.* (1994). Received dose-intensity: a randomized trial of weekly chemotherapy with and without granulocyte colony-stimulating factor in small-cell lung cancer. *Journal of Clinical Oncology* **12**, 77–82

Murray N, Shah A, Osoba D *et al.* (1991). Intensive weekly chemotherapy for the treatment of extensive-stage small-cell lung cancer. *Journal of Clinical Oncology* **9**, 1632–1638

Norton L & Simon R (1977). Tumor size, sensitivity to therapy, and design of treatment schedules. *Cancer Treatment Reports* **61**, 1307–1317

Pettengell R, Woll PJ, O'Connor DA *et al.* (1994). Viability of haemopoietic progenitors from whole blood bone marrow and leukapheresis product: effect of storage media, temperature and time. *Bone Marrow Transplantation* **14**, 703–709

Pettengell R, Woll PJ, Thatcher N *et al.* (1995). Multicyclic, dose intensive chemotherapy supported by sequential reinfusion of haemopoietic progenitors in whole blood. *Journal of Clinical Oncology* **13**, 148–156

Prendiville J, Lorigan P, Hicks F *et al.* (1994) Therapy for small cell lung cancer using carboplatin, ifosfamide, etoposide (without dose reduction), mid-cycle vincristine with thoracic and cranial irradiation. *European Journal of Cancer* **30A**, 2085–2090

Prendiville J, Radford J, Thatcher N *et al.* (1991). Intensive therapy for small-cell lung cancer using carboplatin alternating with cisplatin, ifosfamide, etoposide, mid-cycle vincristine and radiotherapy. *Journal of Clinical Oncology* **9**, 1446–1452

Schabel Jr FM, Griswold Jr DP, Corbett TH, Laster WR (1984). Increasing the therapeutic response rates to anticancer drugs by applying the basic principles of pharmacology. *Cancer* **54**, 1160–1167

Sculier JP, Paesmans M, Bureau G *et al.* (1993). Multiple-drug weekly chemotherapy versus standard combination regimen in small-cell lung cancer: A phase III randomized study conducted by the European Lung Cancer Working Party. *Journal of Clinical Oncology* **11**, 1858–1856

Sheehan RG, Balaban EP, Frenkel EP (1993). The impact of dose intensity of standard chemotherapy regimens in extensive stage small cell lung cancer. *American Journal of Clinical Oncology* **16**, 250–255

Skipper HE (1990). Dose intensity versus total dose of chemotherapy: an experimental basis. In DeVita VT, Hellman S, Rosenberg SA (eds). *Important Advances in Oncology.* Philadelphia: JB Lippincott. pp.43–64

Skipper HE, Schabel Jr FM, Mellett LB *et al.* (1970). Implications of biochemical, cytokinetic, pharmacologic and toxicologic relationships in the design of optimal therapeutic schedules. *Cancer Chemotherapy Reports* **54**, 431–450

Slevin ML, Stubbs L, Plant HJ *et al.* (1990). Attitudes to chemotherapy: comparing views of patients with cancer with those of doctors, nurses, and general public. *British Medical Journal* **300**, 1458–1460

Smith IE, Perren TJ, Ashley SA *et al.* (1990). Carboplatin, etoposide and ifosfamide as intensive chemotherapy for small cell lung cancer. *Journal of Clinical Oncology* **8**, 899–905

Souhami RL, Rudd R, Ruiz de Elvira MC *et al.* (1994). Randomized trial comparing weekly versus 3-week chemotherapy in small-cell lung cancer: a Cancer Research Campaign trial. *Journal of Clinical Oncology* **12**, 1806–13

Steward WP, von Pawel J, Gatzemeier U *et al.* (1998). Effects of granulocyte-macrophage colony-stimulating factor and dose intensification of V-ICE chemotherapy in small-cell lung cancer: a prospective randomized study of 300 patients. *Journal of Clinical Oncology* **16**, 642–50

Taylor CW, Crowley J, Williamson SK *et al.* (1990). Treatment of small-cell lung cancer with an alternating chemotherapy regimen given at weekly intervals: A Southwest Oncology Group Pilot Study. *Journal of Clinical Oncology* **8**, 1811–1817

Tepler I, Elias L, Smith JW *et al.* (1996). A randomized placebo-controlled trial of recombinant human interleukin-11 in cancer patients with severe thrombocytopenia due to chemotherapy. *Blood* **87**, 3607–36

Thatcher N, Girling DJ, Hopwood P (2000). Improving survival without reducing quality of life in small-cell lung cancer patients by increasing the dose intensity of chemotherapy with granulocyte colony stimulating factor support : Results of a British Medical research Council Multicenter Randomised trial. *Journal of Clinical Oncology* **18**, 395–404

Thatcher N, Lind M, Stout R *et al.* (1989). Carboplatin, ifosfamide and etoposide with mid-course vincristine and thoracic radiotherapy for "limited" stage small cell carcinoma of the bronchus.*British Journal of Cancer* **60**, 98–101

Thatcher N, Lorigan P, Burt P, Stout R (1994). Intensive combined modality therapy in small cell lung cancer. *Seminars in Oncology* **21**, 9–23

Trillet-Lenoir V, Green J, Manegold C *et al.* (1993). Recombinant granulocyte colony stimulating factor reduces the infectious complications of cytotoxic chemotherapy. *European Journal of Cancer* **29A**, 319–324

Woll PJ, Hodgetts J, Lomax L *et al.* (1995). Can cytotoxic dose-intensity be increased by using granulocyte colony-stimulating factor? A randomized controlled trial of lenograstim in small-cell lung cancer. *Journal of Clinical Oncology* **13**, 652–9

Woll PJ, Lee SM, Lomax *et al.* (1996). Randomised phase II study of standard versus dose intensive ICE chemotherapy with reinfusion of haemopoietic progenitors in whole blood in small cell lung cancer. *Proceedings of the American Society of Oncology* **15**, 957

Dose intensification of chemotherapy in small cell lung cancer: the case against

Marianne C Nicolson

Introduction

Despite exhibiting impressive chemo-responsiveness, the median survival for patients with small cell lung cancer (SCLC) is appalling, with the majority of patients dying from their disease within 18 months. There has been little improvement in patients' survival over the past twenty years despite study of the use of maintenance therapy, combination of novel drugs and dose intensification of chemotherapy. The latter was first investigated in the 1970s, but poor results prevented the therapy from becoming standard. The lack of benefit seen with high dose therapy in good performance status SCLC patients contrasts with outcomes in other chemosensitive tumours like breast cancer and Hodgkin's disease, and may in part reflect the significant co-morbid disease in lung cancer patients due to their smoking habits. Development of colony stimulating factors and stem cell harvesting, allowing minimisation of the neutropenic period through more rapid repopulation of the bone marrow following high dose chemotherapy, resulted in a renewed enthusiasm for evaluation of the issue of dose intensification of chemotherapy in SCLC. The most troublesome and potentially fatal complication of high dose chemotherapy remains myelosuppression with neutropenic sepsis, but if survival were to be enhanced, the development of second primary cancers is likely to be a problem in this population of smokers. To date, there is scant evidence of any benefit for patients when chemotherapy alone is intensified, as will be demonstrated by the evidence presented below.

Definition of dose intensity

It is known that single agent drug therapy is less effective in SCLC than is combination chemotherapy (Lowenbraun *et al.* 1979). Increasing the number of drugs in a regimen to increase cell kill and perhaps overcome various mechanisms of resistance is one method of intensifying treatment. The actual doses of individual drugs in a regimen may be increased with the therapy still given with the same frequency. Initial high doses of drugs may be administered with subsequent standard doses given. Alternatively, a standard drug combination may be given more frequently – perhaps weekly rather than two- or three-weekly. In the latter situation, bone marrow support is necessary. Means of supporting or 'rescuing' the bone marrow include administration of colony stimulating factors, stem cell rescue or – in the past – autologous bone marrow transplantation.

The different approaches to dose intensification are summarised in Table 10.1.

Table 10.1 Mechanisms of increasing dose intensity

1. Increase number of drugs in regimen
2. Reduce the interval between chemotherapy cycles
3. Increase the dose of individual drugs per cycle, either at initial or all cycles

Dose intensity with standard drug combinations

The most commonly prescribed drug combinations in SCLC include the agents cyclophosphamide, doxorubicin (adriamycin), etoposide, vincristine and platinum (cisplatin or carboplatin). A meta-analysis of the relationship between dose intensity of these drugs in various combinations – cyclophosphamide, adriamycin and vincristine (CAV), cyclophosphamide, adriamycin and etoposide (CAE), cyclophosphamide, adriamycin, vincristine and etoposied (CAVE), etoposide and cisplatin (EP) – and outcome was published by a Canadian group (Klasa *et al.* 1991). In that paper, 60 trials of chemotherapy in SCLC published between 1975 and 1988 incorporating more than 4,500 patients were evaluated for the overall response rates, complete response rate (CR) and median survival (MS) of patients. It was not possible to extract data on one- and two-year survival. Patients with limited disease (LD) and extensive disease (ED) were evaluated separately and intensity was expressed as drug dose administered per meter squared per week. There was no evidence of an improvement in measured outcomes related to increased dose intensity of the first two cycles of chemotherapy. In appreciating that a meta-analysis of retrospective data can serve only to generate a hypothesis for further study, there was no indication here that further investigation of dose intensity would be to the benefit of patients with SCLC.

Increased frequency of dosing

One of the first studies of delivering chemotherapy weekly, as opposed to at the standard three-weekly intervals, was published by the London Lung Cancer Group (Miles *et al.* 1991). The patients had either limited (n=45) or extensive (n=25) SCLC and were of good performance status with favourable biochemical parameters. The authors made the point that these features excluded approximately 70 per cent of patients with extensive disease. Through alternating administration of cisplatin and etoposide or ifosfamide and doxorubicin weekly for a total of 12 weeks, the overall response rate was 91 per cent with 50 per cent CR. MS for the whole group was 54 weeks. The study was extended to randomisation between the same alternating regimens given weekly or three-weekly (Souhami 1994). Despite including 438 patients, there was no significant difference in overall survival or MS. Toxicity in the patients receiving the higher dose resulted in a reduction in dose intensity in the weekly arm, but quality of life was not formally assessed.

A further randomised study of weekly versus standard dosing frequency used adriamycin, etoposide, cyclophosphamide, cisplatin, vindesine, vincristine and methotrexate given in a complex weekly schedule and compared this regimen with adriamycin, cyclophosphamide and etoposide (ACE) (Sculier *et al.* 1993). The 223 patients randomised were reported to have 'tolerable' toxicity but there was increased haematological toxicity in the ACE arm. Despite this, the total relative dose intensity was significantly higher in the ACE arm due to delays in chemotherapy administration in the weekly arm. Five of the six toxic deaths due to neutropenic sepsis were in the weekly treatment arm. There was no significant difference between the two schedules in response or survival.

First cycle dose intensification

Results of studies by the French indicated that increasing the doses of the initial chemotherapy cycle(s) may improve survival for patients with SCLC. They proceeded to a randomised trial in patients with limited disease where the first cycle only of chemotherapy incorporating cisplatin and cyclophosphamide had doses of these drugs increased by 20 and 25 per cent respectively (Arriagada *et al.* 1993). There were 55 patients treated with the higher does and 50 with standard chemotherapy. Concurrent radiotherapy was given to both groups of patients. The surprising outcome was an increase in two-year survival from 26 per cent to 43 per cent in the intensified arm. In a similar randomised trial including 90 chemonaive SCLC patients with extensive disease, treatment was either with high dose etoposide ($80mg/^2$ daily for five days instead of three days in the standard arm) and cisplatin ($27mg/m^2$ days one to five every three weeks as opposed to $80mg/m^2$ day one only) (Ihde *et al.* 1994). Despite the 67 per cent increase in dose for the first two cycles only, the objective response rate and MS were virtually identical, although toxicity was considerably worse in the higher dose patients. The latter authors made the point that the study was small and that only two drugs were given in the combination. However, cisplatin and etoposide is one of the standard regimens in SCLC and the increase in toxicity with no improvement in response would have made extension of the study inappropriate.

The vexing question of the importance of the intensity of the initial doses of chemotherapy in SCLC therefore remains unanswered.

Use of colony stimulating factors to increase dosing frequency

A study of dose intensification in good prognosis patients with SCLC included in one arm addition of granulocyte colony stimulating factor (G-CSF) (Woll *et al.* 1995). The chemotherapy regimen was vincristine, ifosfamide, carboplatin and etoposide (VICE) which is significantly myelosuppressive. Patients received chemotherapy at unfixed intervals, dependent only on their full blood count being adequate for treatment. Sixty-five consecutive patients from a single institution were randomised and, although the white blood cell and neutrophil counts were supported in the G-CSF group, there was no difference in incidence of febrile neutropenia, antibiotic or transfusion requirements. The dose intensity was greater in the G-CSF arm, but the toxic death rate was six compared with only one in the non-intensified group. The two-year survival rate was better in the G-CSF arm – 32 per cent versus 15 per cent – but there was no difference in MS.

The dose interval of the ACE regimen was also reduced to two-weekly from the usual three-weekly cycle through adding G-CSF to reduce the duration of neutropenia (Thatcher *et al.* 1995). The MS was not stated, all 20 patients experienced WHO grade 3 or 4 neutropenia and there were three treatment-related deaths but the regimen was said to be tolerable and was extended to a randomised study discussed later in this chapter. Conversely, in a population of 54 patients with extensive SCLC, accelerated delivery of doxorubicin, etoposide and ifosfamide resulted in severe septic complications, delay in 58 of 244 courses and MS of only eight months (Trillet-Lenoir *et al.* 1996). The authors concluded that the accelerated regimen was too toxic to recommend.

The attempt to increase by 50 per cent the dose intensity of cyclophosphamide, eprubicin, etoposide and cisplatin given monthly with recombinant human GM-CSF (rhGM-CSF) concluded that excessive toxicity in patients with ED SCLC precluded dose intensification (Pujol *et al.* 1997). The controlled arm of the randomised study allocated patients to receive six cycles of standard doses of the same drugs. The cumulative doses were higher in the standard treatment arm, and there was no difference in the response rate. Haematological toxicity was much worse in the intensified arm, and MS was shorter – 8.9 months compared with 10.9 months. Probability of relapse at one year was also increased in the intensified arm – 96 versus 77.

There was similar failure to demonstrate benefit to patients when cisplatin, vincristine, doxorubicin and etoposide (CODE) with g-CSF was compared with CAV-PE in 227 patients with ED SCLC (Furuse *et al.* 1998). There was no significant difference in CR or overall response, MS was 11.6 months for CODE and 10.9 months for CAV-PE. The achieved dose intensity was approximately doubled in the CODE arm and there was more anaemia and thrombocytopenia with CODE. Although there was no difference in leukopenia between the two arms of the study, four patients had a treatment-related death from neutropenic fever with CODE.

Both patients with ED and LD were included in a study where 403 patients were randomised to receive six cycles of either standard three-weekly ACE or two-weekly ACE and G-CSF support (Thatcher *et al.* 2000). This large trial with only one variable – increased frequency of drug delivery using G-CSF – reported an almost identical overall response rate but there was a survival advantage in the intensified arm. At one year, the control group survival was 39 per cent compared with 47 per cent in the intensified arm. The difference was maintained at two years – 8 per cent versus 13 per cent. In this study, there was equivalent advantage in intensifying treatment in patients with ED. There was no difference in toxic death between the standard and the intensified arms of the study, and no negative impact on quality of life was reported by patients who had the two-weekly chemotherapy.

The results of randomised trials of dose intensification with or without colony stimulating factors are summarised in Table 10.2.

Table 10.2 Median survival in randomised studies of dose intensity

Author/year	stage	Number randomised	Median survival Intensified	Standard	CSF?
Souhami, '91	276LD	438	10.8/12	10.6/12	no
Sculier, '93	95LD	223	43/52	49/52	no
Arriagada '93	all LD	105	43%*	26%*	no
Ihde, '94	all ED	90	10.7/12	11.4/12	no
Woll '95	60LD	65	32%*	15%*	yes
Pujol '97	all ED	125	8.9/12	10.8/12	yes
Furuse '98	all ED	227	11.6/12	10.9/12	yes
Thatcher '00	304LD	403	13%*	8%*	yes

*denotes 2-year survival

Late dose intensification

Patients who have demonstrated the chemosensitivity of their SCLC with induction chemotherapy were thought to be those in whom late dose intensification might be appropriate through delivery of very high dose chemotherapy and autologous bone marrow transplant (ABMT).

In his review of studies of ABMT in SCLC, Elias (1998) first evaluated them according to whether patients were untreated, relapsed or refractory, whether they had complete or partial response to first line therapy (CR or PR) and whether extent of disease was LD or ED. Patients were pooled for aggregated relapse free and overall survival characteristics. For the 52 evaluable patients with relapsed or refractory disease, high dose combination chemotherapy did not improve duration of response or survival. The majority of patients (71 per cent) who had initial treatment incorporating ABMT were staged to have LD. Of the 103 patients analysed, the response rate, relapse free, two-year and overall survival were not improved with ABMT. Responding patients who were consolidated with ABMT numbered 282, but despite an increase in CR rate to 50 per cent, there was no overall survival benefit. The mortality rate from the high dose chemotherapy treatment was 18 per cent in one study (Humblet *et al.* 1987), and the lack of improvement in survival lead the investigators in this and other trials to avoid recommendation of the treatment as standard.

Recently, a mature follow-up has been published of a trial where patients with LD or ED SCLC received induction chemotherapy using etoposide, ifosfamide, cisplatin and epirubicin, (VIP-E) followed by peripheral blood stem cell transplant (PBSCT) after high dose etoposide, ifosfamide, carboplatin and epirubicin (VIC-E) conditioning (Fetscher et al. 1999). A total of 100 patients received VIP-E and 30 then proceeded to have VIC-E with PBSCT. Six patients with LD had their tumour surgically resected before chemotherapy started and three of these had induction chemotherapy only. A further five patients had surgery after either induction (four) or high dose (one) chemotherapy. All patients had thoracic radiotherapy. Of the 30 patients who had the high dose therapy, the median survival for patients with ED was eight months and for LD 26 months. Treatment-related mortality was 18 per cent in patients with ED and 10 per cent in patients with LD. There were no survivors at five years in the ED subset, but 33 per cent of the non-resected LD (50 per cent of total LD) patients remained alive. The authors recommended that patients with ED SCLC should not receive the high dose regimen. Of those patients who survived more than two years, 27 per cent developed a second malignancy, and this is a further recognised risk of high dose chemotherapy.

Conclusion

In the review of older and more recent papers presented here, it is clear that, in most studies of intensification of chemotherapy, patients with ED SCLC do not benefit. The aim in these people – most of whom are going to die within a year from their tumour – must remain optimum palliation with combination, standard dose chemotherapy. For the patients of good performance status, favourable biochemistry and LD SCLC, there may be some advantage in giving higher doses in the early treatment cycles, but the evidence is not in favour of this becoming a standard treatment.

It would seem to be much more intelligent – and compassionate – to investigate alternative methods of improving outcomes for these patients, and to abandon the 'more must be better' fixation. The evidence already exists that consolidating the chemotherapy response by giving early consolidation thoracic radiotherapy in responding patients with LD increases survival (Murray et al. 1993). Evaluation of matrix metalloproteinase inhibitors and vaccines are ongoing, and perhaps they will afford benefit without inducing increased toxicity in people with SCLC.

References

Arriagada R, Le Chevallier T, Pignon JP et al. (1993). Initial chemotherapeutic doses and survival in patients with limited small cell lung cancer. *New England Journal of Medicine* **329**, 1848–1852

Elias A (1998). Dose-intensive therapy in small cell lung cancer *Chest* **113**, 101S–106S

Fetscher S, Brugger W, Engelhardt R et al. (1999). Standard- and high-dose etoposide, ifosfamide, carboplatin and epirubicin in 100 patients with small cell lung cancer: A mature follow-up report. *Annals of Oncology* **10**, 561–567

Furuse K, Fukuoka M, Nishiwaki Y *et al.* (1998). phase III study of intensive weekly chemotherapy with recombinant human granulocyte colony stimulating factor versus standard chemotherapy in extensive disease small cell lung cancer. *Journal of Clinical Oncology* **16**, 2126–2132

Humblet Y, Symann M, Bosly A *et al.* (1987). Late intensification chemotherapy with autologous bone marrow transplantation in selected small cell carcinoma of the lung: A randomised study. *Journal of Clinical Oncology* **5**, 1864–1873

Ihde DC, Mulshine JL, Kramer BS *et al.* (1994). Prospective randomised comparison of high dose and standard dose etoposide and cisplatin chemotherapy in patients with extensive stage small cell lung cancer. *Journal of Clinical Oncology* **12**, 2022–2034

Klasa RJ, Murray N, Coldman AJ (1991). Dose-intensity meta-analysis of chemotherapy regimens in small-cell carcinoma of the lung *Journal of Clinical Oncology* **9**, 499–508

Lowenbraun S, Bartolucci A, Smalley RV *et al.* (1979). The superiority of combination chemotherapy over single agent chemotherapy in small cell lung carcinoma. *Cancer* **44**, 406–413

Miles DW, Earl HM, Souhami RL *et al.* (1991). Intensive weekly chemotherapy for good prognosis patients with small cell lung cancer. *Journal of Clinical Oncology* **9**, 280–285

Murray N, Coy P, Pater JL *et al.* (1993). Importance of timing for thoracic irradiation in the combined modality treatment of limited stage small cell lung cancer. *Journal of Clinical Oncology* **11**, 336–44

Pujol J-L, Douillard J-Y, Riviere A *et al.* (1997). Dose-intensity of a four grug chemotherapy regimen with or without recombinant human granulocyte macrophage stimulating factor in extensive stage small celll lung cancer: A multicenter randomised phase III study. *Journal of Clinical Oncology* **15**, 2082–2089

Sculier JP, Paesmans M, Bureau G *et al.* (1993). Multiple drug weekly chemotherapy versus standard combination regimen in small cell lung cancer: A phase III randomised study conducted by the European Lung Cancer Working Party. *Journal of Clinical Oncology* **11**, 1858–1865

Souhami RL, Rudd R, Ruiz de Elvira M–C *et al.* (1994). Randomised trial comparing weekly versus 3-week chemotherapy in small-cell lung cancer: a Cancer Research Campaign trial. *Journal of Clinical Oncology* **12**, 1806–13

Thatcher N, Anderson H, Bleehen NM *et al.* (1995). The feasibility of using glycosylated recombinant human granulocyte colony-stimulating factor (G-CSF) to increase the planned dose intnesity of doxorubicin, cyclophosphamide, and etoposide (ACE) in the treatment of small cell lung cancer. *European Journal of Cancer* **31A**, 152–156

Thatcher N, Girling DJ, Hopwood P *et al.* (2000). Improving survival without reducing quality of life in small cell lung cancer patients by increasing the dose intensity of chemotherapy with granulocyte colony-stimulating factor support: Results of a British Medical Research Council multicenter randomised trial. *Journal of Clinical Oncology* **18**, 395–404

Trillet-Lenoir V, Soler P, Arpin D *et al.* (1996). The limits of chemotherapy dose intensification using granulocyte colony stimulating factor alone in extensive small cell lung cancer. *Lung Cancer* **14**, 331–341

Woll PJ, Hodgetts J, Lomax L *et al.* (1995). Can cytotoxic dose intensity be increased by using granulocyte colony stimulating factor? A randomised controlled trial of Lenograstim in small cell lung cancer. *Journal of Clinical Oncology* **13**, 652–659

Chapter 11

The evidence base for palliative chemotherapy

Graham G Dark and Mary O'Brien

Introduction

Non-small cell lung cancer (NSCLC) accounts for about 80 per cent of all primary lung cancers, and 60 per cent of cases present as advanced stages IIIB and IV disease. There is a median survival of four–six months without treatment and only 10–20 per cent of patients can be expected to be alive at one year (NSCLC Collaborative Group 1995). Despite the widespread use of palliative chemotherapy for other cancers, there continues to be a reluctance to prescribe chemotherapy for advanced NSCLC. The early studies of chemotherapy demonstrated limited success with no clear survival benefit and many clinicians had a view that chemotherapy was unjustified for anyone not in a clinical trial (Haskell 1991). However, in recent years, the introduction of platinum containing regimens has produced modest improvements in survival and additional studies have demonstrated that chemotherapy can significantly improve the quality of life and control symptoms in many patients with advanced disease.

Prognostic factors for response and survival

Several important prognostic factors have been identified, which have the potential to affect both response and survival and which must be considered when evaluating the usefulness of combination chemotherapy (Table 11.1). The most important prognostic determinant of survival and response rate is the stage or extent of disease. Patients with locally advanced disease have higher response rates when compared to those seen when the same regimen is administered to patients with bone marrow metastases (Ray *et al.* 1998). Metastatic deposits in the liver or bone are less likely to respond than those in the lung, subcutaneous or lymphatic tissues. Response rates are higher

Table 11.1 Important prognostic factors in the treatment of non-small cell lung cancer with chemotherapy

Factors that significantly affect response	*Factors predictive of survival*
M1 stage disease	M1 stage disease
Performance status	Performance status
Involvement of liver, bone, bone marrow	Pre-treatment weight loss
Use of combination chemotherapy	Elevated lactate dehydrogenase
	Female sex

when comparing combination chemotherapy with single-agent treatment, particularly if the combination regimen includes cisplatin, a vinca alkaloid, mitomycin C, or ifosfamide (Bakowski & Crouch 1983; Joss *et al.* 1984; Haskell 1991).

Other factors associated with poor survival include a lack of objective response to chemotherapy, presence of metastasis, poor performance status, pre-treatment weight loss, and an elevated LDH (Albain *et al.* 1991), whereas age and histological subtype have not consistently been shown to correlate with either response or survival (Sakurai *et al.* 1987; Bonomi *et al.* 1991; Lee & Hong 1992; Feld *et al.* 1994; Ray *et al.* 1998; Van Zandwijk & Van't Veer 1998).

Most of the published trials of chemotherapy for patients with stage IIIB or IV disease have included patients with performance status (ECOG 0-2), as poor performance status correlates with an increased risk of severe toxicity and early death (Ruckdeschel *et al.* 1986). This finding has been confirmed in a retrospective audit, by the authors, of all patients with NSCLC referred to a medical oncologist and that subsequently received chemotherapy over a five-year period at the Royal Marsden Hospital. This study included 590 patients and defined early death as death occurring within 21 days of receiving chemotherapy, i.e., from either progressive disease or toxicity. Overall, the early death rate was 8.5 per cent. There was no sex or age correlation, but the most important factor predictive of early death was performance status. The early death rates for patients with NSCLC receiving chemotherapy are outlined in Table 11.2. The study group had a median age of 65; 83.9 per cent of patients were receiving first-line therapy and 13.5 per cent were receiving second-line. The results indicate a steep increase in risk of early death with chemotherapy as the performance status of the patient deteriorates. Thus chemotherapy should only be offered to patients in relatively good condition, noting that age is not a risk factor (Hickish *et al.* 1995). Future chemotherapy may have fewer adverse effects or toxicity and may allow the use of agents in poor condition patients, but the risk of death due to toxicity may be greater than the likelihood of symptomatic benefit and requires careful investigation. The current COIN guidelines suggest a toxic death rate of less than 10 per cent as a standard, and these data may provide evidence of what is achievable and contribute to the future recommendations.

Assessment of outcomes of palliative chemotherapy

Although response rates and survival are standard criteria against which any treatment is assessed, palliation of symptoms can occur in the absence of conventionally defined criteria for response to treatment. There are several studies which show that, despite a low objective response rate of around 30 per cent, up to 70 per cent of patients report relief of symptoms when treated with modern chemotherapy (Hardy *et al.* 1989; Ellis *et al.* 1995; Cullen *et al.* 1999).

The assessment of toxicity associated with chemotherapy has been objective, often by using the Common Toxicity Criteria, which facilitates comparison between

Table 11.2 Early deaths occurring within 21 days of chemotherapy administration for NSCLC at the Royal Marsden Hospital, stratified by ECOG performance status

Performance status	No. patients	Early deaths (%)
PS 0	41	0.0
PS 1	220	5.5
PS 2	179	10.1
PS 3	54	25.9
PS 4	1	100.0
Unknown	95	5.3

different trials, but this fails to accurately assess the subjective improvements or the impact of a particular side effect upon the individual, and thus gauge the patient's experience of the treatment. There is a need to include this subjective data in addition to the objective criteria and it is hoped that measurements of quality of life will fulfil this need. Quality of life (QoL) reflects a number of elements including physical, psychological, cognitive, social, emotional and economic well-being. There are a number of instruments available for the assessment of QoL, disease- and treatment-related symptoms and their significance to the patient.

There are a number of difficulties relating to QoL research published to date. The most significant problem is that many studies either did not incorporate the information into the trial design or the quality of the data collected was insufficient, compounded by a lack of agreed criteria for reporting (Montazeri *et al.* 1998). Furthermore, although many of the reports documented the toxicities of chemotherapy that may have produced adverse effects on QoL, few have adequately analysed the beneficial effects of chemotherapy on symptom control and overall palliation.

Therefore, work in this area must address a number of problems. There is no standard instrument in use that would allow direct comparison between trials or participating centres (Hopwood *et al.* 1998). The interpretation of the patients symptoms differs depending on who is making the assessment (Hopwood & Stephens 1995; Hopwood 1996). Furthermore, there are no standardised time points for assessing QoL, and almost 30 per cent of patients drop out at the time of their second assessment (Stephens *et al.* 1999). Clinicians involved in this work must be familiar with using QoL data in research studies, but as yet there is no evidence that it should be used as an integral part of the decision-making process in the day-to-day management of patients. Finally, a considerable volume of QoL data has been published, but because of inconsistencies and the heterogeneous nature of the data, statisticians have been quick to criticise this aspect of the research (Stephens *et al.* 1999).

Quality of life research is critical for the evaluation of new therapies, since many patients would not choose chemotherapy for its likely survival benefit of three months, but that they would choose it if it improved QoL (Silvestri *et al.* 1998).

Whilst waiting for the science of QoL to develop, patients with lung cancer get penalised, by denying then both standard and new therapies.

Effects of chemotherapy on survival

The usefulness of chemotherapy in advanced disease continues to be a controversial issue as response rate alone is an inadequate measure of the usefulness of combination chemotherapy. Patients who respond to chemotherapy are more likely to live longer than those who do not, but chemotherapy only contributes a modest improvement to the survival of treated patients with advanced NSCLC (approximately 2–3 months increase in median survival) (NSCLC Collaborative Group 1995). The first studies of non-platinum chemotherapy showed no benefit and indeed some showed a worse outcome in the treatment group (Green *et al.* 1969). More recently a number of clinical trials in advanced NSCLC have been undertaken that prospectively randomised between chemotherapy plus best supportive care versus best supportive care alone. These data from randomised phase III studies are summarised in Table 11.3 (Cormier *et al.* 1982; Rapp *et al.* 1988; Ganz *et al.* 1989; Buccheri *et al.* 1990; Woods *et al.* 1990; Cellerino *et al.* 1991; Kaasa *et al.* 1991; Quoix *et al.* 1991; Leung *et al.* 1992; Cartei *et al.* 1993; Perrone *et al.* 1998; Thatcher *et al.* 1998; Cullen *et al.* 1999; Thongprasert *et al.* 1999).

Unfortunately, much of this trial data is heterogeneous, with response rate varying between 8 and 42 per cent and including stages IIIB and IV. Some included only T4 tumours or cytology positive pleural effusions as stage IIIB and others included mediastinal disease. This is an important issue as stage is the most important prognostic determinant of survival, and patients with stage IIIB disease have a greater survival with chemotherapy than those with stage IV disease (Woods *et al.* 1990).

In the first series by Cormier *et al.* (1982), a highly significant difference in survival was found, but this study is unique in that it randomised to placebo rather than best supportive care and enrolled only 39 patients. This result has been criticised because of the relatively short survival of the control arm (Ganz *et al.* 1989). However, a significant fact was that radiotherapy was not permitted during the trial, possibly accounting for the observed short median survival in the control group of 8.5 weeks. The same trial design was used for a repeat study, but radiotherapy was permitted in both groups and the best supportive care arm had a median survival of 20 weeks (Buccheri *et al.* 1989). The repeat trial confirmed a survival benefit for chemotherapy but, more importantly, it suggested that the inclusion of radiotherapy in best supportive care may bias the effectiveness. This effect of radiotherapy is also suggested in the study by Ganz *et al.* (1989), where the control group, of best supportive care only, had longterm survivors (>55 months) and many of the patients received radiotherapy doses exceeding 40Gy, producing a response rate of 12 per cent in the control arm. Thus the inclusion of radiotherapy as a supportive care treatment may confound the more recent survival data (Anderson *et al.* 2000). Moreover it

Table 11.3 Chemotherapy versus best supportive care in randomised studies in locally advanced or metastatic NSCLC

Reference	Patients	Regimen	Response rate (%)	Median survival (weeks)	p value
(Cormier et al. 1982)	39	MACC placebo	35 –	30.5 8.5	0.0005
(Rapp et al. 1988)	150	CAP VP BSC	15.3 25.3 –	24.7 32.6 17	0.05 0.01
(Ganz et al. 1989)	48	VP BSC	22 12	20.4 13.6	0.09
(Buccheri et al. 1990)	175	MACC BSC	8 –	32 20	0.01
(Woods et al. 1990)	188	VP BSC	28 –	27 17	0.33
	stage IIIB only	VP BSC	– –	45 26	0.075
(Cellerino et al. 1991)	128	CEP/MEC BSC	21 –	34.3 21.1	0.153
(Kaasa et al. 1991)	87	PE BSC	11 –	22.1 16.5	0.29
(Quoix et al. 1991)	49	VP BSC	41.7 –	28.4 10.4	<0.001
(Leung et al. 1992)	119	PE BSC	21 –	49 34	0.047
(Cartei et al. 1993)	102	PCM BSC	25 –	34 16	0.001
(Perrone et al. 1998)	161	V BSC	20 –	25 19	0.04
(Thatcher et al. 1998)	157	T BSC	15 –	27 19	0.045
(Cullen et al. 1999)	351	MIC BSC	32 –	26 19	0.03
(Thongprasert et al. 1999)	287	IEP MVP BSC	40 41.7 –	23 32 16	0.0003

Key: BSC: best supportive care; MACC: methotrexate, doxorubicin, cyclophosphamide, CCNU; CAP: cyclophosphamide, doxorubicin, cisplatin; VP: vindesine, cisplatin; CEP/MEC: cyclophosphamide, epirubicin, cisplatin alternating with methotrexate, etoposide, CCNU; PE: cisplatin, etoposide; PCM: cisplatin, cyclophosphamide, mitomycin C; MIC: mitomycin C, ifosfamide, cisplatin; V: vinorelbine; T: paclitaxel illustrates the fact that there has been little consistency about the definition of best supportive care within the published clinical trials.

A number of meta-analyses of these data have been performed and confirm a survival benefit for chemotherapy against best supportive care, of between two–three months (Souquet *et al.* 1993, 1995; Marino *et al.* 1994; NSCLC Collaborative Group 1995). The meta-analysis by the non-small cell collaborative group assessed the randomised trials that used supportive care plus chemotherapy versus supportive care (11 trials, 1,190 patients) and confirmed the significant heterogeneity both between trials and between chemotherapy categories ($p=0.003$) (NSCLC Collaborative Group 1995). For the eight cisplatin based trials the hazard ratio was 0.73 (95 per cent CI: 0.63,0.85, $p<0.0001$). The results for longterm alkylating agents suggested a detrimental effect, but there were only two trials and the result was not significant. Hazard ratio=1.26 (95 per cent CI: 0.96,1.66, $p=0.095$). Subgroup analyses were undertaken for cisplatin-based regimens only and no evidence of any differences was found. The overall duration of chemotherapy varied in the studies and the criteria for dose reduction and discontinuation were often not clearly defined.

Single agent navelbine is effective and well tolerated in the elderly, producing a significant survival advantage ($p= 0.03$) and increase in median survival from 21 to 28 weeks (Gridelli *et al.* 1997; ELVIS Group 1999). Gemcitabine and taxol as single agents have also been compared to best supportive care and show improved survival, symptom control and QoL (Thatcher *et al.* 1995, Ranson & Thatcher 1999). Chemotherapy doublets have been studied, with gemcitabine compared to cisplatin-etoposide, which showed equivalence for survival. However, the single agent produced a greater probability of achieving a tumour response after two months, with less clinical and haematological toxicity and a significant worsening of symptomatology in the cisplatin/etoposide arm for hair loss, nausea and vomiting, and appetite loss (ten Bokkel Huinink *et al.* 1999). Another study showed that the addition of cisplatin to vinorelbine, compared to single agent vinorelbine produces a higher response rate and a longer survival duration suggesting that doublets may be advantageous (Le Chevalier *et al.* 1994). Gemcitabine-cisplatin versus mitomycin C, ifosfamide, cisplatin showed an improved response rate (38 per cent versus 26 per cent), but no significant difference in survival or time to progression. Crino *et al.* (1999) demonstrated no improvement in QoL for gemcitabine-cisplatin but, nevertheless, gemcitabine-cisplatin is now considered standard therapy in some countries.

Second line therapy with docetaxel for patients with advanced NSCLC who demonstrate platinum-resistant disease can produce a three to four month increase in median survival and one year survival of 40 per cent (Fossella & Rigas 1999). This compares to the use of second-line irinotecan in advanced colon cancer (Cunningham & Glimelius 1999; Ranson & Thatcher 1999), but nevertheless the acceptance of second-line palliative treatment is greater for colon than lung cancer.

Effects of chemotherapy on symptoms and quality of life

Many of the trials of palliative chemotherapy in advanced NSCLC documented the toxicities that may have produced adverse effects on QoL, but few analysed the beneficial effects of chemotherapy on symptom control and overall palliation and omitted objective measurement of QoL.

There is evidence that palliative chemotherapy in advanced NSCLC can improve patients performance status. A study at the Royal Marsden Hospital showed a tumour response rate of 21 per cent using MVP (mitomycin C, vinblastine and cisplatin) for patients with advanced disease (Hardy *et al.* 1989). However, 75 per cent of patients receiving chemotherapy had complete resolution or significant improvement of at least one of their tumour-related symptoms at a single time point, with an overall symptom response rate of 67 per cent. A follow up report with greater patient numbers demonstrated an overall response rate of 32 per cent, but patients with locally advanced disease (stage IIIB) had a significantly better response rate (52 per cent) than those with metastatic disease (25 per cent) (*p*< 0.01). Reflecting the improved objective response rate in stage IIIB patients, 78 per cent of patients with locally advanced disease had resolution or substantially improved symptoms (69 per cent overall). Symptomatic improvement was achieved after one course of chemotherapy in 61 per cent and after two courses in 96 per cent of responding patients (Ellis *et al.* 1995).

Most of the trials of palliative chemotherapy against supportive care have focused on response rates and duration of survival as measures of outcome, and data from these studies on the duration of chemotherapy is heterogeneous. No significant benefit has been demonstrated by increasing the treatment duration. Moreover, a trial of MVP chemotherapy showed that three courses produced the same symptomatic benefits and response rates as six, but had significantly less toxicity (Smith *et al.* 1998).

Several other studies utilising platinum-based chemotherapy combinations have shown that responses in symptoms can be demonstrated even in the absence of objective tumour responses, and that up to 70 per cent of patients report relief of symptoms when treated with modern chemotherapy (Fernandez *et al.* 1989; Hardy *et al.* 1989; Anderson *et al.* 1994; Ellis *et al.* 1995; Montazeri *et al.* 1998; Cullen *et al.* 1999; ELVIS Group 1999) (Anderson *et al.* 2000).

Economic analysis of palliative chemotherapy

The economic implications of palliative treatment for advanced NSCLC may be substantial as there is a perception that chemotherapy is expensive and, in view of the modest survival gain in the magnitude of weeks, is not cost-effective. However, economic evaluation in a Canadian study has demonstrated that the majority of cost is related to hospitalisation and not to the use of chemotherapy agents (Jaakkimainen *et al.* 1990). This compares favourably with estimates of cost-effectiveness of commonly used treatments for other diseases and emphasises that a policy of supportive care is associated with costs that may exceed those of active treatment.

Although the randomised trials of chemotherapy have only demonstrated modest survival gains, a review of 17 studies that utilised data from various sources to model the impact and cost of chemotherapy showed that chemotherapy for stages IIIB and IV NSCLC can be cost-effective and, in some cases, may actually be less expensive than supportive care alone (Mather *et al.* 1998). Economic analysis of chemotherapy in various studies has indicated cost-effectiveness for a number of drug combinations (Evans 1993; Evans & Le Chevalier 1996; Earle & Evans 1999; Kelly 1999). Furthermore, these studies indicate that allocating resources for chemotherapy in this setting can be justified relative to many treatment expenditures for other types of cancer and other disease. Moreover, economic evaluation of inoperable non-small-cell lung cancer can provide important information to complement survival and quality-of-life data in resource allocation decisions (Mather *et al.* 1998). Currently, most of the data relating to economic analysis is Canadian or French and there is a need for data from the United Kingdom, which should be available in due course from the Big Lung Trial.

Conclusions

There is good evidence that chemotherapy is beneficial in the palliation of advanced NSCLC, but when patients have disseminated metastases present, chemotherapy will never be curative, and both the patient and the physician must understand that palliation is the objective of treatment. To this end, when reporting chemotherapy trials, investigators should be encouraged to include an assessment of QoL, to determine whether the toxicity of treatment is balanced not only by prolongation of life, but also by a reduction in symptoms, thus producing palliation.

Whenever possible, patients should be treated in clinical trials of either new agents or new combinations of drugs. Continued assessment of new drugs and novel treatment strategies in patients with advanced disease is essential to identify regimens that may have sufficient activity to justify their future use in patients with earlier stages of lung cancer. This has become the case over the last five years in the management of breast, prostate and colon cancer. The remaining questions for chemotherapy for advanced NSCLC are whether triplets of agents are superior to doublets or single agents, whether new drugs with less side effects can increase survival and improve QoL. There are a number of ongoing studies to answer these issues. Furthermore, in the UK, extra resources in terms of appropriately trained specialists with interest and enthusiasm are required to contribute to the research and development of this field (O'Brien & Cullen 2000).

Widespread nihilism towards chemotherapy has meant that patients with all stages of lung cancer may have been deprived of treatment that adds small survival gains. This in turn may contribute to the dismal outcome survival figures for lung cancer in the UK. At this time chemotherapy is sufficiently active to justify its use in patients of good performance status who understand the true goals of chemotherapy and its potential toxicities.

References

Albain KS, Crowley JJ, LeBlanc M *et al.* (1991). Survival determinants in extensive-stage non-small-cell lung cancer: the Southwest Oncology Group experience. *Journal of Clinical Oncology* **9**, 1618–26

Anderson H, Hopwood P, Stephens RJ *et al.* (2000). Gemcitabine plus best supportive care (BSC) versus BSC in inoperable non-small cell lung cancer – a randomised trial with quality of life as the primary outcome. *British Journal of Cancer* **83**, 447–453

Anderson H, Lund B, Bach F *et al.* (1994). Single-agent activity of weekly gemcitabine in advanced non-small-cell lung cancer: a phase II study. *Journal of Clinical Oncology* **12**, 1821–6

Bakowski MT and Crouch JC (1983). Chemotherapy of non-small cell lung cancer: a reappraisal and a look to the future. *Cancer Treatment Reviews* **10**, 159–72

Bonomi P, Gale M, Rowland K *et al.* (1991). Pre-treatment prognostic factors in stage III non-small cell lung cancer patients receiving combined modality treatment. *International Journal of Radiation Oncology, Biology, Physics* **20**, 247–52

Buccheri GF, Ferrigno D, Curcio A *et al.* (1989). Continuation of chemotherapy versus supportive care alone in patients with inoperable non-small cell lung cancer and stable disease after two or three cycles of MACC. Results of a randomized prospective study. *Cancer* **63**, 428–32

Buccheri G, Ferrigho D, Rosso A *et al.* (1990). Further evidence in favor of chemotherapy for inoperable non-small cell lung cancer. *Lung Cancer* **6**, 87

Cartei G, Cartei F, Cantone A *et al.* (1993). Cisplatin-cyclophosphamide-mitomycin combination chemotherapy with supportive care versus supportive care alone for treatment of metastatic non-small-cell lung cancer. *Journal of the National Cancer Institute* **85**, 794–800

Cellerino R, Tummarello D, Guidi F *et al.* (1991). A randomized trial of alternating chemotherapy versus best supportive care in advanced non-small-cell lung cancer. *Journal of Clinical Oncology* **9**, 1453–61

Cormier Y, Bergeron D, La Forge J *et al.* (1982). Benefits of polychemotherapy in advanced non-small-cell bronchogenic carcinoma. *Cancer* **50**, 845–9

Crino L, Scagliotti GV, Ricci S *et al.* (1999). Gemcitabine and cisplatin versus mitomycin, ifosfamide, and cisplatin in advanced non-small-cell lung cancer: A randomized phase III study of the Italian Lung Cancer Project. *Journal of Clinical Oncology* **17**, 3522–30

Cullen MH, Billingham LJ, Woodroffe CM *et al.* (1999). Mitomycin, ifosfamide, and cisplatin in unresectable non-small-cell lung cancer: effects on survival and quality of life. *Journal of Clinical Oncology* **17**, 3188–94

Cunningham D & Glimelius B (1999). A phase III study of irinotecan (CPT-11) versus best supportive care in patients with metastatic colorectal cancer who have failed 5-fluorouracil therapy. V301 Study Group. *Seminars in Oncology* **26**, 6–12

Earle CC & Evans WK (1999). Cost-effectivenes of paclitaxel plus cisplatin in advanced non-small-cell lung cancer. *British Journal of Cancer* **80**, 815–20

Ellis PA, Smith IE, Hardy JR *et al.* (1995). Symptom relief with MVP (mitomycin C, vinblastine and cisplatin) chemotherapy in advanced non-small-cell lung cancer. *British Journal of Cancer* **71**, 366–70

ELVIS Group (1999). Effects of vinorelbine on quality of life and survival of elderly patients with advanced non-small-cell lung cancer. *Journal of the National Cancer Institute* **91,** 66–72

Evans WK (1993). Management of metastatic non-small-cell lung cancer and a consideration of cost. *Chest* **103,** 68s–71s

Evans WK & Le Chevalier T (1996). The cost-effectiveness of navelbine alone or in combination with cisplatin in comparison to other chemotherapy regimens and best supportive care in stage IV non-small cell lung cancer. *European Journal of Cancer* **32a,** 2249–55

Feld R, Borges M, Giner V *et al.* (1994). Prognostic factors in non-small cell lung cancer. *Lung Cancer* **11,** S19–23

Fernandez C, Rosell R, Abad Esteve A *et al.* (1989). Quality of life during chemotherapy in non-small cell lung cancer patients. *Acta Oncology* **28,** 29–33

Fossella FV & Rigas J (1999). The use of docetaxel (Taxotere) in patients with advanced non-small cell lung cancer previously treated with platinum-containing chemotherapy regimens. *Seminars in Oncology* **26,** 9–12

Ganz PA, Figlin RA, Haskell CM *et al.* (1989). Supportive care versus supportive care and combination chemotherapy in metastatic non-small cell lung cancer. Does chemotherapy make a difference? *Cancer* **63,** 1271–8

Green RA, Humphrey E, Close H *et al.* (1969). Alkylating agents in bronchogenic carcinoma. *American Journal of Medicine* **46,** 516–25

Gridelli C, Perrone F, Gallo C *et al.* (1997). Vinorelbine is well tolerated and active in the treatment of elderly patients with advanced non-small cell lung cancer. A two-stage phase II study. *European Journal of Cancer* **33,** 392–7

Hardy JR, Noble T, Smith IE (1989). Symptom relief with moderate dose chemotherapy (mitomycin-C, vinblastine and cisplatin) in advanced non-small cell lung cancer. *British Journal of Cancer* **60,** 764–6

Haskell CM (1991). Chemotherapy and survival of patients with non-small cell lung cancer. A contrary view [editorial]. *Chest* **99,** 1325–6

Hickish TF, Smith IE, Ashley S *et al.* (1995). Chemotherapy for elderly patients with lung cancer [letter]. *Lancet* **346,** 580

Hopwood P (1996). Quality of life assessment in chemotherapy trials for non-small cell lung cancer: are theory and practice significantly different? *Seminars in Oncology* **23,** 60–4

Hopwood P & Stephens R J (1995). Symptoms at presentation for treatment in patients with lung cancer: implications for the evaluation of palliative treatment. The Medical Research Council (MRC) Lung Cancer Working Party. *British Journal of Cancer* **71,** 633–6

Hopwood P, Harvey A, Davies J *et al.* (1998). Survey of the Administration of quality of life (QL) questionnaires in three multicentre randomised trials in cancer. The Medical Research Council Lung Cancer Working Party the CHART Steering Committee. *European Journal of Cancer* **34,** 49–57

Jaakkimainen L, Goodwin PJ, Pater J *et al.* (1990). Counting the costs of chemotherapy in a National Cancer Institute of Canada randomized trial in nonsmall-cell lung cancer. *Journal of Clinical Oncology* **8,** 1301–9

Joss RA, Cavalli F, Goldhirsch A *et al.* (1984). New agents in non-small cell lung cancer. *Cancer Treatment Reviews* **11,** 205–36

Kaasa S, Lund E, Thorud E *et al.* (1991). Symptomatic treatment versus combination chemotherapy for patients with extensive non-small cell lung cancer. *Cancer* **67,** 2443–7

Kelly K (1999). The role of single-agent gemcitabine in the treatment of non-small-cell lung cancer. *Annals of Oncology* **10,** S53–6

Le Chevalier T, Brisgand D, Douillard JY *et al.* (1994). Randomized study of vinorelbine and cisplatin versus vindesine and cisplatin versus vinorelbine alone in advanced non-small-cell lung cancer: results of a European multicenter trial including 612 patients. *Journal of Clinical Oncology* **12**, 360–7

Lee JS & Hong WK (1992). Prognostic factors in lung cancer [editorial]. *New England Journal of Medicine* **327**, 47–8

Leung WT, Shiu WC, Pang JC *et al.* (1992). Combined chemotherapy and radiotherapy versus best supportive care in the treatment of inoperable non-small-cell lung cancer. *Oncology* **49**, 321–6

Marino P, Pampallona S, Preatoni A *et al.* (1994). Chemotherapy vs supportive care in advanced non-small-cell lung cancer. Results of a meta-analysis of the literature. *Chest* **106**, 861–5

Mather D, Sullivan SD, Parasuraman TV (1998). Beyond survival: economic analyses of chemotherapy in advanced, inoperable NSCLC. *Oncology Huntingt* **12**, 199–209

Montazeri A, Gillis CR, McEwen J (1998). Quality of life in patients with lung cancer: a review of literature from 1970 to 1995. *Chest* **113**, 467–81

NSCLC Collaborative Group (1995). Chemotherapy in non-small cell lung cancer: a meta-analysis using updated data on individual patients from 52 randomised clinical trials. Non-small Cell Lung Cancer Collaborative Group. *British Medical Journal* **311**, 899–909

O'Brien MER & Cullen M (2000). Guidelines must help bring us in line with European standards [letter]. *British Medical Journal* **320**, 1604

Perrone F, Rossi A, Ianniello GP *et al.* (1998). Vinorelbine plus best supportive care versus best supportive care in the treatment of advanced non-small cell lung cancer elderly patients. Results of a phase III randomised trial. *Proceedings of the American Society of Clinical Oncology* **17**, 455a

Quoix E, Dietemann A, Charbonneau J *et al.* (1991). Is chemotherapy with cisplatin useful in non small cell bronchial cancer at staging IV? Results of a randomized study. *Bulletin of Cancer* **78**, 341–6

Ranson M & Thatcher N (1999). Paclitaxel: A hope for advanced non-small cell lung cancer? *Expert Opinion on Investigational Drugs* **8**, 837–848

Rapp E, Pater JL, Willan A *et al.* (1988). Chemotherapy can prolong survival in patients with advanced non-small-cell lung cancer—report of a Canadian multicenter randomized trial. *Journal of Clinical Oncology* **6**, 633–41

Ray P, Quantin X, Grenier J *et al.* (1998). Predictive factors of tumor response and prognostic factors of survival during lung cancer chemotherapy. *Cancer Detection and Prevention* **22**, 293–304

Ruckdeschel JC, Finkelstein DM, Ettinger DS *et al.* (1986). A randomized trial of the four most active regimens for metastatic non-small-cell lung cancer. *Journal of Clinical Oncology* **4**, 14–22

Sakurai M, Shinkai T, Eguchi K *et al.* (1987). Prognostic factors in non-small cell lung cancer: multiregression analysis in the National Cancer Center Hospital (Japan). *Journal of Cancer Research and Clinical Oncology* **113**, 563–6

Silvestri G, Pritchard R and Welch HG (1998). Preferences for chemotherapy in patients with advanced non-small cell lung cancer: descriptive study based on scripted interviews. *British Medical Journal* **317**, 771–5

Smith IE, O'Brien MER, Norton A *et al.* (1998). Duration of chemotherapy for advanced non-small cell lung cancer (NSCLC): A phase III randomised trial of 3 versus 6 courses of Mitomycin C, Vinblastine, Cisplatin (MVP). *Proceedings of the American Society of Clinical Oncology* **17**, 457a

Souquet PJ, Chauvin F, Boissel JP *et al.* (1995). Meta-analysis of randomised trials of systemic chemotherapy versus supportive treatment in non-resectable non-small cell lung cancer. *Lung Cancer* **12**, S147–54

Souquet PJ, Chauvin F, Boissel JP *et al.* (1993). Polychemotherapy in advanced non small cell lung cancer: a meta-analysis. *Lancet* **342**, 19–21

Stephens RJ, Hopwood P, Girling DJ (1999). Defining and analysing symptom palliation in cancer clinical trials: a deceptively difficult exercise. *British Journal of Cancer* **79**, 538–544

ten Bokkel Huinink WW, Bergman B, Chemaissani A *et al.* (1999). Single-agent gemcitabine: an active and better tolerated alternative to standard cisplatin-based chemotherapy in locally advanced or metastatic non-small cell lung cancer. *Lung Cancer* **26**, 85–94

Thatcher N, Anderson H, Betticher DC *et al.* (1995). Symptomatic benefit from gemcitabine and other chemotherapy in advanced non-small cell lung cancer: changes in performance status and tumour-related symptoms. *Anticancer Drugs* **6**, 39–48

Thatcher N, Ranson M, Anderson H (1998). phase III study of paclitaxel versus best supportive care in inoperable non-small cell lung cancer. *Annals of Oncology* **9**, 1

Thongprasert S, Sanguanmitra P, Juthapan W *et al.* (1999). Relationship between quality of life and clinical outcomes in advanced non-small cell lung cancer: best supportive care (BSC) versus BSC plus chemotherapy. *Lung Cancer* **24**, 17–24

Van Zandwijk N & Van't Veer LJ (1998). The role of prognostic factors and oncogenes in the detection and management of non-small-cell lung cancer. *Oncology Huntingt* **12**, 55–9

Woods RL, Williams CJ, Levi J *et al.* (1990). A randomised trial of cisplatin and vindesine versus supportive care only in advanced non-small cell lung cancer. *British Journal of Cancer* **61**, 608–11

PART 5

Multidisciplinary intervention and the development of effectiveness and efficiency in service delivery

Management of breathlessness in advanced lung cancer: new scientific evidence for developing multidisciplinary care

Jessica Corner

Introduction

To date much of the research conducted to date into lung cancer has concentrated on oncological treatment, yet lung cancer causes many difficult and debilitating symptoms that have a negative impact on quality of life and function. Pain, weight loss, breathlessness and cough are common and often are not relieved. Research into the problems patients experience as a result of having lung cancer is limited, as are studies into the best strategies for alleviating or managing these. This deficiency reflects the fact that symptom management for this disease is currently poorly understood and is not always given priority in care or treatment settings.

While pain is common in lung cancer, occuring in around 50 per cent of patients at presentation (Muers & Round 1993; Hopwood & Stephens 1995), and in as many as 80 per cent of patients admitted to palliative care units (Krech *et al.* 1992), in general it is less common and more readily alleviated than respiratory problems such as breathlessness and cough. Studies of the symptoms experienced by people with lung cancer indicate that 75 per cent may report breathlessness at diagnosis or when first attending for treatment (Muers & Round 1993; Stevens & Firth 1992). In a needs assessment study undertaken on behalf of Macmillan Cancer Relief, more than 80 per cent of 209 patients with lung cancer who completed a postal questionnaire reported breathlessness as a problem. Breathlessness was also reported by patients' GPs as the most challenging aspect of their work with lung cancer (Krishnasamy & Wilkie 1999).

Studies of patients in the last weeks of life suggest that breathlessness may be intractable or poorly treated. In one study of patients following referral to a specialist palliative care team, breathlessness, unlike pain which improved very early in care, was not controlled at all (Higginson & McCarthy 1989). A study of patients attending the MD Anderson Cancer Centre in Texas (Escelente *et al.* 1996) found that breathlessness was the fourth most common reason for attendance in the emergency department, occurring in 80 per cent of those admitted. Patients admitted from the emergency department as a result of breathlessness had a median stay in hospital of nine days and 25 per cent had more than one visit to the emergency department as a result of breathlessness. These data suggest that, even in a specialist cancer hospital, breathlessness is a significant problem for patients and symptom control is poor, resulting in costly health care interventions.

Little research has been undertaken into the problem of breathlessness in lung cancer or into strategies for managing the symptom. Brown *et al.* (1986) interviewed 80 people diagnosed with lung cancer who also reported shortness of breath. In describing breathlessness, 'difficult breathing', 'hard to move air' and 'tired' or 'frightened', were used in addition to reporting 'shortness of breath'. Feelings of suffocation were also common. As well as the symptom itself, breathlessness was said to cause poor concentration, memory loss and sweating. The symptom had severely limited the activity of patients, leaving 80 per cent of those interviewed feeling socially isolated. While these patients had found strategies for managing their breathlessness, such as modifying their activities, slowing down and accepting the situation, worryingly, only 10 per cent of those interviewed had received any help or advice on how to cope with breathlessness from health professionals.

A study by Roberts *et al.* (1993) of patients with breathlessness in late stage cancer revealed that only 39 per cent of patients had any record of the problem made in their medical or nursing notes. Interviews with nurses caring for them revealed great inconsistencies over their understanding of the symptom and the extent to which it was felt to be a problem, thus giving the impression that breathlessness may go unreported and unrecognised. One nurse commented that, because patients intuitively limit activity in response to breathlessness, the problem becomes invisible to health professionals. It appeared that patients did not generally report breathlessness, while at the same time health professionals did not consider it a priority for intervention or help.

Treatment for breathlessness in advanced cancer has been focused on the use of chemotherapy, radiotherapy and procedures such as drainage of pleural effusions (Cowcher & Hanks 1990). If it is not possible to reverse the cause of breathlessness, pharmacological interventions, such as opioids or anxiolytics are used to alleviate the symptom (Davis *et al.* 1996; Boyd & Kelly 1997). Other therapies such as nebulised drugs, corticosteroids, acupuncture and other complementary therapies have also been used. However, little evidence exists for the effectiveness of these treatments.

The potential contribution of nursing to the management of breathlessness has not, as yet, been fully recognised. Nurses have developed an important role in the management of breathlessness in chronic pulmonary disease and asthma, and some services in these areas are nurse-led. While in these situations the role of nursing is well established, this is not the case in breathlessness as a result of advanced cancer. In response to this, the author and a team of nurse researchers from the Centre for Cancer and Palliative Care Studies at the Institute of Cancer Research, have developed and evaluated a nursing approach to managing breathlessness in lung cancer in a series of studies.

Managing breathlessness: a nursing perspective

Previously strategies employed in managing breathlessness in advanced cancer, and more particularly lung cancer, have taken a biomedical approach. That is to say the focus has been on the pathophysiology of breathlessness, although this is poorly understood. In lung cancer the approach has been to use treatments such as radiotherapy to reduce the size of tumours that may be occluding airways, or where a patient has a plueral effusion, to drain it. In advanced cancer, the perspective of palliative care has been to see breathlessness as irreversible and therefore not amenable to cause directed treatment. Instead, the symptom has been understood as a nociceptive problem and therefore similar to pain. Treatment is aimed at removing or reducing the sensation of breathlessness centrally and morphine and/or an anxiolytic is prescribed. Research into the palliation of breathlessness has largely focused on pharmacological treatments, and the few studies undertaken have evaluated different modes of delivering such treatment, for example via a nebuliser (Davis *et al.* 1996). Other treatments have been evaluated, such as oxygen (Bruera *et al.* 1993; Booth *et al.* 1996) and acupuncture (Filshie 1996). In all cases the results have been equivocal (Department of Health 1998). Inadequate study designs have been employed, and very small samples of patients used. As a result of this inadequate research, it is difficult to determine whether treatments are ineffective or poor study designs have prevented the detection of a treatment effect that may exist. In any event, it would appear that the management of breathlessness needs a new approach.

In developing a nursing approach it seemed that strategies used to date failed to address some fundamental aspects of the problem of breathlessness in lung cancer namely:

- the current recognition that, for the majority, lung cancer is incurable and treatment directed at the tumour is unlikely to reverse the problem of breathlessness. Therefore a model of symptom management based on cure or containment of the disease itself is unlikely to be effective, except temporarily;
- the palliative care approach too readily assumes that it is possible to remove the sensation of breathlessness using pharmacological means. Also, it employs the strongest pharmacological tools at the outset (i.e., opioids), without trying other strategies first. Thus, although the approach is modelled on well established methods of pain control, cardinal rules regarding its management (i.e., the analgesic staircase) are broken;
- an understanding of cancer symptoms which acknowledges that these occur in the context of an integrated mind and body has not been adopted in mainstream treatment and care. Therefore the contribution of emotions such as fear, anxiety or depression to the symptom experience is neglected. There is also a failure to acknowledge that breathlessness in lung cancer is experienced in the face of incurable, indeed imminently life threatening, illness;

- despite a growing literature on respiratory rehabilitation for chronic respiratory disease and asthma, techniques used in these contexts have been overlooked in breathlessness associated with advanced cancer. In particular it is surprising that the need to adapt one's life to this disabling condition has not been recognised or addressed.

The nursing approach, listed below, was developed to incorporate a number of the features felt to be missing in existing symptom management strategies.

- An integrative model, in which the emotional experience of breathlessness is considered inseparable from the sensory experience and from the pathopysiological mechanisms, was adopted. Each component of the factors that contribute to breathlessness was considered equally important. The use of this integrative approach led to the adoption of a model of care used in parallel to conventional biomedical approaches (see Figure 12.1). The model is rehabilitative in its orientation and care is directed at assisting individuals to manage the problem of breathlessness for themselves, rather than for the symptom to become solely the object of the health professional's ministrations.
- Intervention is primarily delivered in the context of a nurse-led outpatient clinic. In the clinic, care is less dominated by an institutional environment, patients attend voluntarily and bring family members or friends to the consultation should they wish. A reciprocal relationship between patient and nurse is developed and breathlessness is viewed as a problem in which both patient and nurse have a mutual interest. Ways of managing breathlessness are therefore discovered together. The nurse is therapist, but the object of therapy, breathlessness, is the subject of mutual enquiry by both patient and nurse. The relationship is therefore one of equality. Care is focused on agreeing goals whereby improved function or episodes of breathlessness may be achieved, which are then reviewed at subsequent clinic visits.
- The importance of encouraging and listening to the patient's story of their illness and how breathlessness is experienced as part of this is recognised, and is a central part of intervention. Clinic sessions with nurses begin with a form of assessment, this largely consisting of the facilitation of an ongoing narrative, or story telling, regarding illness and breathlessness. Here the team is influenced by Kleinman's (1988) notion of ' illness narratives' and the therapeutic potential in working with such narratives. A clinical assessment tool has been developed to facilitate assessment interviews about the problem of breathlessness, based on the approach developed by the team (Corner & O'Driscoll 1999). Formal measures of breathlessness, such as visual analogue scales, are also used to record change in self-ratings of the symptom over time.

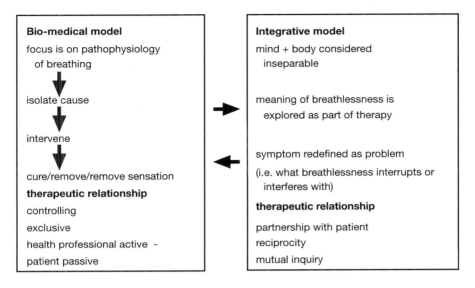

Figure 12.1 Parallel models of breathlessness management

- Fundamental to the approach is the recognition that much of what is therapeutic in listening to patients' stories of their breathlessness is hearing and 'holding' fear and distress associated with the symptom. Bailey (1995), in describing the nursing approach as 'therapy', draws on Bion (1962) and Fabricius (1991) to explain the process of therapeutic work: the nurse makes herself available, psychically, as a container for anxieties that are intolerable. This is a maternal function whereby, like a mother with an infant, intolerable stress is contained and processed, and in time fed back in a tolerable form. The primal link between breathing and life, ceasing to breathe and dying, is frequently central to fear of breathlessness and may itself evoke or exacerbate attacks of the symptom. Often patients quite literally fear they will die during their next episode of breathlessness, yet often have never voiced this fear. For others the association is less manifest, yet the triggers for episodes of breathlessness share these associations. For example, one man attending the clinic reported that the onset of his breathlessness followed the moment the curtains were drawn across his mother's coffin during the committal at her funeral. Another man found his breathlessness commenced in the evening on drawing the curtains of his bedroom and that, as a result, he preferred to sleep in a chair in the sitting room in order to avoid it. Other associations with previous experiences unfold often in apparently disconnected ways during recounting of stories such as wartime experiences, twins that were stillborn two decades earlier, a sister dying of the same condition. In exploring experiences together, the aim is to assist patients to understand how and why such associations and fears arise, and that these are not in themselves real. Realisation that breathlessness in itself is not life threatening and that fears and associations may arise as a result of facing lung cancer, can help mitigate some of the disabling effects of breathlessness since activity may be limited as a result of fears and beliefs about breathlessness. Hearing sadness, anger or frustration arising from illness or knowledge of having an incurable illness may also be therapeutic.

- Intervention employs a number of techniques derived from respiratory rehabilitation, such as breathing re-training, energy conservation, life adaptation, and, for breathlessness in the more advanced stages of illness, relaxation and distraction techniques. Breath re-training involves teaching breathing control techniques. This aims to correct an unconscious tendency for people suffering from breathlessness to breathe in rapid short breaths from their upper chest using the accessory respiratory muscles. Instead, lower chest breathing at a relaxed, normal rate is taught, as are methods for adopting this pattern while walking or climbing stairs or during episodes of breathlessness. Using lower chest breathing reduces effort and is thought to move air in and out of the lungs more effectively as well a promoting gas exchange. Learning to adapt one's life and activities to the problems imposed by breathlessness is a central part of intervention.

- The integrative model is realised in practice through a complex balancing of practical assistance and facilitation of adjustment to the limitations imposed by breathlessness, with explicit and implicit recognition of the distress and fear of that accompanies the symptom. As Bailey (1995) states:

> 'there is scope for developing nursing roles within a framework that makes it possible to be more accepting of patients' "conscious and unconscious demands", to employ nursing as therapy. The order of nursing situations; the routine; the way in which "symptoms" are dealt with at a high level of abstraction; the prevalence of models or algorithms which "stand for" human entities without expressing them; the splitting of human experience into neatly bound categories, setting aside the undisciplined whole; all of this stands in the way, provides a means to become detached, to leave painful things untouched. If nursing can change these things, the opportunities are unlimited.'

Evaluating the effectiveness of nursing intervention for breathlessness

Nursing intervention has been evaluated in a series of studies. First, a small pilot study was undertaken at the Royal Marsden Hospital (Corner *et al.* 1996). Thirty-four patients with small cell and non-small cell lung cancer, who had completed chemotherapy or radiotherapy and reported breathlessness, consented to take part in a randomised study comparing nursing intervention with standard care.

Patients randomised to the intervention group attended weekly sessions with a nurse research practitioner, each session lasting approximately one hour, using the approach already outlined. Further follow-up sessions were available if required. The control group received detailed assessments of their breathlessness during outcome assessment interviews. They were encouraged to talk freely about their breathlessness but were not offered breathing re-training or counselling. Outcomes were assessed using visual analogue scales to rate breathlessness over the past week, functional capacity and the Hospital Anxiety and Depression Scale (Zigmond & Snaith 1983). In depth interviews were conducted to explore the experience of breathlessness. Both groups were assessed on entering the study, at four weeks and at three months.

Although 14 patients had to withdraw from the study due to illness progression and death, leaving 20 patients for the analysis, the results were promising. Analysis of data showed median scores for breathlessness at best and at worst, distress caused by breathlessness, functional capacity and difficulty in performing activities of daily living, reduced over time in the intervention group. Using Wilcoxon tests, the differences observed were significant. In the intervention group ratings of distress improved by a median of 53 per cent and there was a median improvement in functional capacity of 17 per cent. In contrast the median scores for the control group were static or worsened over time. Comparison of change scores between the two groups revealed significant improvements for the intervention group in visual analogue scale ratings of breathlessness, functional capacity and ability to perform activities of daily living.

Interviews with patients in the control group revealed the depth of distress and the enormous limitation caused by breathlessness. Over time patients reported relinquishing all activity, episodes of panic were common and feelings of loss were expressed as they experienced life as increasingly limited by breathlessness. In contrast the intervention group described increasing activity and functional levels by using breathing control techniques. Patients reported managing to control episodes of panic, pace themselves and achieve goals. They found the opportunity to talk with a nurse valuable and reported expanding their horizons again provided they paced themselves, acknowledged their physical limitations, and addressed fears. Although the study appeared to indicate that the nursing approach was effective it was small and therefore conclusions drawn from it limited.

A second study was conducted in parallel with the pilot evaluation of the intervention, and is reported by O'Driscoll et al. (1999). It was originally intended that 60 patients would be recruited. However, after 34 patients had been randomised to the pilot evaluation, randomisation was stopped in response to requests by medical and nursing staff who felt they had observed a clear benefit from the intervention strategy. The remaining 26 patients were offered, and attended for, nursing intervention.

On first entering the study, and at each subsequent visit to the nursing clinic, or at four weeks and three months for patients in the control group, the nurse researcher completed a semi-structured assessment with the patient. Details of the patient's disease, stage and treatment, understanding of their illness, social circumstances, current concerns and goals, were recorded during or immediately following conversations concerning patients' descriptions of their breathlessness, their emotional responses to it, the effect it had on their lives and any self help strategies they used. The assessment notes were then analysed using a form of content analysis. Data from 52 of these assessment notes were sufficiently complete for use in the analysis.

The assessment notes revealed powerful images used to describe breathlessness and how it influenced every part of the person's life. It was difficult to separate physical and non-physical aspects of breathlessness since these were intricately woven together in the language used. For example, one patient's description of their breathlessness was:

'…you don't think you'll get it back again-like suffocation, frightened the life out of me…breath is more important than water.'

Another description of breathlessness emphasised the deeply emotional nature of the symptom and the association of breathlessness with dying:

'…when the shortness of breath was at its extreme, I thought I was going to die and saw a coffin beside me and then I was in a tunnel…I did have thoughts about suicide and I envied the dead…'

Fear and panic were common emotions associated with breathlessness. Panic was recorded as part of breathlessness for 21 (40 per cent) of the patients, and the feeling of impending death for 16 (31 per cent).

Contrary to the common assumption that breathlessness is experienced continuously by patients with lung cancer, only eight (15 per cent) of patients reported this. For the remaining 44 (85 per cent) it was more intermittent in character. Patients described attacks of breathlessness that lasted from minutes up to an hour, although attacks lasted between 5 and 15 minutes for the majority. Attacks of breathlessness were commonly associated with a triggering factor such as physical exertion. Walking, climbing stairs, or carrying heavy objects triggered breathlessness in 52 per cent of patients; activities such as washing, dressing, housework or shopping triggered it in 19 per cent; changing positions such as bending or standing up in 17 per cent; activities involving the oral/respiratory tract such as eating, talking or drinking in 17 per cent and environmental factors such as a cold wind in 15 per cent of patients. Emotions were reported to trigger breathlessness in 13 per cent of patients. For example one woman said:

'…if I talk too much I get out of breath, if I walk too much I get out of breath, if I walk to the shop or lift anything I loose my breath, or if I get cross or emotional, shopping – by the time I get to the check out, I have had enough – I hold on to the trolley for support, dressing is a bit of a bind, getting out of the bath, going up stairs – I'm breathless at the top, housework – I need to rest between activities and I don't do any hard housework…'

The finding that breathlessness was intermittent and triggered by events or activities for the majority was important. It confirmed the researchers' view that taking a rehabilitative approach, whereby assistance is directed at the activities interrupted or interfered with by breathlessness, rather than aimed at alleviating the symptom itself, was correct, especially since the most commonly used palliative treatment, morphine, is generally reserved for those who have continuous breathlessness while at rest. Breathlessness had imposed restrictions on life for those suffering from it in both managing activities inside the house and in carrying on work or, for example, gardening. Social activities and sexual relations were also affected. For many, the symptom contributed to feelings of uncertainty and hopelessness about the future. The cost of breathlessness to family members and carers was also apparent: one man recounted the very distressing experience of watching his wife dying while suffering from unrelieved breathlessness, and his feelings of helplessness. Acknowledging the restrictions imposed by breathlessness and trying to find ways of adjusting to these or making adaptations to one's life to minimise them, as well as involving family members in learning ways of coping with breathlessness, was as a result of this study, incorporated into the nursing intervention approach.

Following the success of the pilot evaluation, a third study was undertaken to replicate this with a larger sample of patients and to assess whether it was possible to translate the intervention approach into other settings around the UK. A multicentre randomised controlled trial of nursing intervention for breathlessness in patients with lung cancer was undertaken, funded by Macmillan Cancer Relief, as part of the work of the Institute of Cancer Research's Macmillan Practice Development Unit. The findings are reported by Bredin *et al.* (1999). Macmillan and specialist cancer nurses in six UK centres established nurse-led clinics for breathlessness management with the help and support of the Macmillan Practice Development Unit. A similar study design was used as in the pilot evaluation. Patients with both small cell and non-small cell lung cancer and mesothelioma, who had completed treatment and reported breathlessness, were invited to take part in the study. Randomisation was independent. Intervention was offered to patients allocated to the treatment group by Macmillan and specialist nurses in the participating centres using the nursing approach. Patients attended the nursing clinic once a week for up to eight weeks (and for not less than three weeks). The control group was offered standard care for breathlessness. Data were collected from both groups at weeks one, four and eight. Outcome measures included visual analogue scales measuring breathlessness at worst and at best and distress due to breathlessness, WHO performance status scale, the Hospital Anxiety and Depression Scale and the Rotterdam Symptom Checklist.

One hundred and nineteen patients were recruited to the study. One centre failed to adhere to the trial protocol, and data for its 16 patients were excluded on the advice of the data monitoring committee. Sixteen patients died during the course of the study and 28 patients withdrew. The most common reason for withdrawing was because the patient's condition deteriorated. No appreciable difference in medication was found between the two groups and therefore this did not appear to account for the effects seen.

For the analysis, at the outset of the study the principal time point selected for assessing outcome was from baseline to eight weeks when the intervention was believed to have had maximum effect. Patients withdrawing from the study, other than those who reported being too well to continue, were given a change score that was one more (that is, worse) than the maximum of patients who did not withdraw. Those who reported being too well to continue were given a score which was one less than the minimum score of those who did not withdraw, as recommended by Gould (1980). The Mann-Whitney test was used to assess differences in change scores between the two groups.

At baseline, the data revealed high levels of distress and functional impairment among the patients. At eight weeks, the intervention group showed significant improvement in ratings of breathlessness at best ($p=0.03$), performance status ($p=0.02$), levels of depression ($p=0.02$) and physical symptom distress ($p=0.04$). Levels of anxiety ($p=0.08$) and ratings of distress due to breathlessness ($p=0.09$) improved less. The findings of the study thus appear to confirm those of the pilot study, and suggest that patients with breathlessness associated with lung cancer benefit from attending clinics using the nursing approach.

The nursing contribution to the problem of breathlessness in lung cancer

Through the programme of research the team of nurses working at the Institute of Cancer Research believe that significant progress has been made in understanding and assisting patients in managing the difficult and distressing symptom of breathlessness. A series of studies have been undertaken, including detailed analysis of the experience of breathlessness in 52 patients with lung cancer. Further data from the 119 patients who took part in the multicentre clinical trial is currently being analysed. A new model of working with breathlessness, based on a non-pharmacological and self-management approach, and considering the fears associated with breathlessness, has been developed. This has been piloted in a small single centre trial which indicated that the approach was effective. The results were replicated in a multicentre randomised controlled trial in six centres throughout the UK. The challenge now is to ensure that the approach is widely adopted. A new study has been initiated from the Macmillan Practice Development Unit which aims to disseminate the approach and investigate methods of ensuring that it is used in practice.

Centres where there are nurse specialists in lung cancer are being invited to become, with the help of the Unit, teaching and demonstration centres to foster and pass on good practice in the management of breathlessness. The Macmillan Practice Development Unit is developing teaching materials to support the resource centres using a variety of different media such as a web site, an interactive CD ROM and a textbook. The work of the resource centres will be supported through a network of practitioners facilitated by the Unit. It is intended that the dissemination project will be evaluated using collaborative inquiry methods.

Treatment for lung cancer and the symptoms associated with it has traditionally been seen as medical territory, although this has been accompanied by attitudes which have had negative consequences for quality of care. In order to improve treatment and care in the future it is now recognised that a multidisciplinary approach is needed. Nurses will increasingly play an important role in the management of patients with lung cancer. The programme of research into breathlessness has demonstrated the value of a more inclusive approach. Nurses have brought a fresh view to a difficult problem and taken the initiative in demonstrating its value. A similar strategy may prove fruitful for other problems associated with lung cancer and, if so, much larger strides in enhancing the quality of life for the many people suffering from this difficult disease, may be made.

References

Bailey C (1995). Nursing as therapy in the management of breathlessness in lung cancer. *European Journal of Cancer Care* **4**, 184–190

Bion W (1962). Learning from experience. In *Seven Servants*. Jason Aronson, New York

Booth S, Kelly MJ, Cox NP, Adams L, Guz A (1996). Does oxygen help dyspnea in patients with cancer. *American Journal of Respiratory Critical Care Medicine* **153**, 1515–1518

Boyd KJ & Kelly M (1997). Oral morphine as symptomatic treatment of dyspnoea in patients with advanced cancer. *Pallitaive Medicine* **11**, 277–281

Bredin M, Corner J, Krishnasamy M, Plant H, Bailey C, A'Hern R (1999). Multicentre randomised controlled trial of nursing intervention for breathlessness in patient with lung cancer. *Bristish Medical Journal* **318**, 901–904

Brown ML, Carrieri V, Janson- Bjerklie SJ, Dodd SJ (1986). Lung cancer and dyspnea: the patient's perception. *Oncology Nursing Forum* **13**, 519–524

Bruera EN, de Stoutz A, Velasco-Leiva T, Schoeller T, Hanson J (1993). Effects of oxygen on dyspnea in hypoxaemic terminal-cancer patients *Lancet* **342**, 13–14

Corner J, Plant H, A'Hern R, Bailey C, (1996). Non-pharmacological intervention for breathlessness in lung cancer. *Palliative Medicine* **10**, 29–305

Corner J & O'Driscoll M (1999). Development of a breathlessness assessment guide for use in palliative care. *Palliative Medicine* **13**, 375–384

Cowcher K & Hanks GW (1990). Long-term management of respiratory symptoms in advanced cancer. *Journal of Pain and Symptom Management* **5**, 320–330

Davis C, Penn K, A'Hern R, Daniels J, Slevin M (1996). Single dose randomised controlled trial of nebulised morhpine in patients with cancer related breathlessness. *Palliative Medicine*. Research abstract, **10**, 64–5

Department of Health (1998). *NHS Executive, Guidance on Commissioning Services: Improving Outcomes of Lung Cancer*. London:Department of Health

Escelente CP, Martin CG, Elting LS, Cantor SD (1996). Dyspnea in cancer patients, etiology, resource utilisation and survival – implications in a managed care world. *American Cancer Society* **78**, 1314–1319

Fabricius J (1991). running on the spot or can nursing really change. *Psychoanalytic Psychotherapy* **5**, 97–108

Filshie J (1996). Acupuncture for the relief of cancer-related breathlessness. *Palliative Medicine* **10**, 145–150

Gould A L (1980). A new approach to the analysis of clinical drug trials with withdrawals. *Biometrics* **36**,721–7

Higginson I & McCarthy M (1989). Measuring symptoms in terminal cancer: are pain and dyspnoea controlled? *Journal of the Royal society of Medicine* **82**, 264–7

Hopwood P & Stevens RJ (1995). Symptoms at presentation for treatment of patients with lung cancer: implications for evaluation of palliative treatment. The Medical Research Council Lung Cancer Working Party. *British Journal of Cancer* **71**, 633–636

Kleinman A (1988). The Illness Narratives: Suffering, Healing and the Human Condition. New York: Basic Books

Krech R, Davis J, Walsh D (1992). Symptoms of lung cancer. *Palliative Medicine* **6**, 309–315

Krishnasamy M & Wilkie E (1999). *Lung Cancer: Patient's and Families' and Professionals' Perceptions of Health Care Need. A National Needs Assessment Study*. Unpublished research report. London: Macmillan Practice Development Unit, Institute of Cancer Research

Muers MF & Round CE (1993). Palliation of symptoms in non-small cell lung cancer: a study by thr Yorkshire Regional Organisation Thoracic Group. *Thorax* **48**, 339–343

O'Driscoll M, Corner J, Bailey C (1999). The experience of breathlessness in lung cancer. *European Journal of Cancer Care* **8**, 37–43

Roberts DK, Thorne S E, Pearson C (1993). The experience of dyspnea in late stage cancer: patients' and nurses perspectives. *Cancer Nursing* **16**, 234–236

Stevens G & Firth I (1992). Non-small cell lung carcinoma of th elung a retrospective study. *Australaisan Radiobiology* **36**, 243–248

Zigmond AS & Snaith RP (1983). The hospital anxiety and depression scale. *Acta Psychiatrica Scandinavica* **67**, 361–370

Chapter 13

The development and implementation of clinical practice guidelines in the development of an effective service

Peter Simmonds

Introduction

Lung cancer is an important clinical problem, being the most common cancer in the United Kingdom and also the leading cause of cancer death, accounting for around 37,000 deaths each year (Cancer Research Campaign 1996). The effective management of patients with lung cancer is dependent upon both the process by which care is provided, ensuring rapid and accurate diagnosis and staging, as well as the quality of the treatment and supportive care provided. Evidence from up-to-date, good quality research should underpin the management of this common problem. However, there is increasing recognition that care of individuals and delivery of services to populations responds slowly and unevenly to new research evidence (Haines & Jones 1994), and that important advances, well supported by evidence, may take years to become adopted (Ketley & Woods 1993). There is also evidence that both between (Berrino *et al.* 1995) and within (Maher *et al.* 1993) countries, there is greater variation in clinical practice and outcomes than can be justified by case mix alone. Such differences suggest that clinicians use different information to inform treatment decisions.

Health care professionals are under increasing pressure to ensure that practice is evidence-based, since this is perceived to support the development of best practice and improve the quality of patient care. Traditional methods of continuing medical education and scientific publication have been ineffective in promoting the incorporation of research evidence into clinical practice (Davis *et al.* 1995; Freemantle *et al.* 1997). Guidelines enable health professionals to access information on clinical effectiveness and can achieve changes in clinical practice or organisation (Karjalainen & Palva 1989; Grimshaw & Russell 1993; Winstanley *et al.* 1995; Haynes *et al.* 1997). In order to utilise guidelines appropriately, it is necessary to understand what they are, how they are developed, what their limitations are and how they are best implemented.

What are guidelines?

Clinical practice guidelines are systematically developed statements that assist clinicians and patients in making decisions about appropriate treatment for specific conditions (West & Newton 1997). Guidelines attempt to distil a large body of evidence into a convenient, readily usable format (Eddy 1990). The formulation of guidelines thus involves gathering, appraising, and combining evidence. Guidelines go beyond most overviews in attempting to address all the issues relevant to a clinical decision and all the value judgements about the relative importance of various health and economic outcomes in specific clinical situations (Hayward *et al.* 1995).

What is the purpose of guidelines?

The central role of guidelines is to help clinicians make better decisions. They are aids to, not substitutes for, clinical judgement. They can improve the process of health care and health outcomes by making evidence-based standards explicit and accessible, thereby decreasing practice variation and optimising the use of resources (Audet *et al.* 1990; Pearson *et al.* 1995). When based on a synthesis of the most valid and current research evidence, clinical practice guidelines for diseases such as lung cancer can help health professionals keep up-to-date with the literature and help them assimilate evidence into practice (Greengold & Weingarten 1996). The process of care will thereby be improved and clinical decision making will be more objective.

In addition to this central role, the development of guidelines may have other benefits. When suitably repackaged, guidelines can play a role in helping to inform and empower patients. Examining primary research and published reviews in preparation for guideline formulation often identifies gaps in medical knowledge where the research evidence is insufficient to inform management decisions. This can be a powerful stimulus for future research. Guidelines and recommended pathways of care can also provide the ideal structure for effective audit (West & Newton 1997) by identifying practical measures that help users to audit their performance against guideline recommendations.

Guideline development

Increasing attention is being paid to the methodology of guideline development, as there is a relationship between the methodology used to prepare guidelines and the validity of their recommendations. Recommendations based on rigorous methods are associated with greater validity than those based on informal ones (Grimshaw *et al.* 1995a). Although judgements are always involved to some degree, good methodology makes the rationale behind recommendations transparent and understandable to users (Haward 1998).

All of the health professionals likely to play an important role in the implementation of clinical practice guidelines should be involved in their development (Haward 1998), to ensure that professional influence is broad-based. Patient and carer perspectives are also increasingly being considered, despite difficulties or biases in securing such representation. Jackson and Feder (1998) have identified three important steps in guideline development. The key to developing usable guidelines is to identify the most important clinical decisions in patient management. These generally relate to making a diagnosis, estimating prognosis, assessing relevant outcomes, including the risks, benefits and costs of alternative treatments, and weighing up the various consequences of different treatment options. Unless guidelines are limited to major decision points they become too unwieldy to use in practice. The second component of successful guidelines is bringing together the relevant, valid evidence that clinicians need to make informed decisions at each of the key decision points. Guidelines based on an incomplete evaluation of the literature can lead to inappropriate recommendations: the search for relevant research should be comprehensive, research should be selected using explicit criteria and the validity of the results should be judged in a rigorous and reproducible fashion. Guideline developers should ideally search for, select, critique and combine data in a manner analogous to that used for a systematic review.

Although guideline developers are increasingly able to access comprehensive and systematic overviews of the evidence related to specific clinical questions, this does not remove the need for at least some critical appraisal of the original studies in order to understand the populations, interventions, and outcomes evaluated, the heterogeneity of these features and individual study results. Not all outcomes of interest are measured in all primary studies. Thus, certain measures, such as quality of life, are often inadequately represented in reviews. Randomised trials are often underpowered for rare events or unusual adverse effects of treatment and may not report them, so systematic reviews may not provide such information.

In addition to incorporating evidence and acknowledging its absence, creating clinical recommendations requires making value judgements about preferred courses of action in specific clinical situations. The strength of treatment recommendations is ideally informed by the quality of the research evidence, the magnitude, precision, and reproducibility of the treatment effect and the relative value (determined by guideline developers, health care workers and patients) of various outcomes. The prospective development and application of a systematic approach to appraising and classifying evidence is important because this means that the strength of the evidence in support of recommendations can be reported, making the background to individual statements clear to users. By providing clear rankings of the level of evidence used to inform guideline decisions and correlating this with the strength of the recommendation, guideline users are made aware of the basis for the recommendations and the extent to which the recommendations reflect the strength of the research evidence. Wilson *et al.* (1995) have also suggested that guideline developers should undertake a sensitivity analysis by considering the possibility that the effect of a management option on an outcome, or the relative value of different outcomes, is much greater, or much less, than their best estimate. This might be useful in highlighting the uncertainty of many of the estimates on which recommendations are based.

The third essential component of a successful guideline is the presentation of evidence and recommendations in a concise, accessible format (Jackson & Feder 1998). Practice guidelines are usually presented in a framework congruent with decision making to enable users to retrieve and assimilate information quickly. Moreover, the information should be presented in a format that is applicable to specific patients or circumstances.

All guidelines lose force as new evidence emerges after publication that may qualify or even contradict published recommendations. Feedback from users may also suggest weaknesses in the original document that could be remedied in a subsequent version. Periodic review and amendment of guidelines is part of good methodology (Haward 1998).

Assessment of clinical practice guidelines

Concern has been raised about the quality, reliability and independence of some practice guidelines (Grilli *et al.* 2000). Users therefore need to assess the strengths and weaknesses of any given guideline through evaluation of the contents against explicit criteria (Cluzeau *et al.* 1999). Several authors have highlighted key issues in the appraisal of clinical practice guidelines (Hayward *et al.* 1995; Wilson *et al.* 1995; Greenhalgh 1997). Primarily this involves assessing the validity of the recommendations made in the guidelines and determining whether they will be helpful in patient care. Three principal factors may influence guideline validity: the composition of the guideline group (encompassing the range of disciplines and proportion of guideline users involved), methods of synthesising evidence and the process of developing guidelines (Grimshaw *et al.* 1995a).

The strength of guideline recommendations should be informed by multiple considerations, including the quality of the research that provided the evidence for the recommendations, the magnitude and consistency of positive outcomes relative to negative outcomes (adverse effects, burdens to the patient, and health care system costs), and the relative value placed on different outcomes (Wilson *et al.* 1995). Determining the validity of the recommendations involves assessing whether all reasonable management options and all important potential outcomes have been considered and whether appropriate methods were used to find and appraise all the relevant data relating to the recommendations made. It is important to determine whether and how expert opinion was used to fill in gaps in the evidence from clinical trials. If there is no information about how treatment options and outcomes were chosen, how evidence was selected and how values were established, it is not possible to evaluate whether these steps have been performed systematically and such guidelines may not be valid (Hayward *et al.* 1995).

For many clinical questions there is frequently inadequate evidence, and thus a variety of studies have to be considered, as well as reports of expert and consumer experience (Hayward *et al.* 1995). It is important that there is a clear link between the strength of recommendations and the quality and quantity of evidence on which they are based. A quality of evidence scale is often used to rate different categories of evidence and the methods for producing it, according to the likelihood that the results will be biased. Such classification systems usually emphasise that the strongest evidence comes from rigorous randomised controlled trials and weaker evidence from observational studies using cohort or case control designs. Inferring strength of evidence from study design alone may overlook other factors that determine the quality of the evidence such as sample size, recruitment bias, losses to follow up, unmasked outcome assessment, atypical patient groups, unreproducible interventions and atypical clinical settings (Wilson *et al.* 1995). Moreover, the results from a single randomised controlled trial with a small sample size are not necessarily more convincing than consistent results with large precision from a large number of high quality trials of non-randomised design conducted in a variety of places and times (Wilson *et al.* 1995). Overviews should filter out studies with major design flaws and, if meta-analysis is performed, the precision, magnitude, and heterogeneity of study results should be considered (Wilson *et al.* 1995). Guidelines based on randomised controlled trials are stronger when the results of individual studies are similar, and weaker when major differences between studies (heterogeneity) are present (Wilson *et al.* 1995). If guidelines are developed on the basis of observational studies, or if the estimate of the treatment effect is imprecise, strong recommendations should not be expected unless major harms and costs are associated with the intervention, or a catastrophic outcome (e.g., death) may be prevented by a low-risk, low-cost intervention of probable efficacy (Wilson *et al.* 1995).

In answering many health care questions, important strands of evidence may come from observational and population-based studies, audit and grey literature. Even then, significant gaps in knowledge may be apparent which make the task of guideline development difficult. Haward (1998) has identified common weaknesses in the research evidence base for cancer services. These include: organisation of services, such as the contribution of the multidisciplinary team members and benefits of centralisation; resolving relationships between individual expertise, specialisation and caseload to outcomes; evaluating the impact of various elements of multi-modality treatment on outcome; defining optimal surgical management; management of advanced or recurrent disease; quantifying patient needs and economic studies relating costs to service patterns or effectiveness.

The clinical problems for which guidelines are most needed often involve complex trade-offs between competing benefits, harms and costs, and are associated with considerable uncertainty (Hayward *et al.* 1995). Even in the presence of strong evidence from randomised clinical trials, the effect size of an intervention may be marginal, or the intervention may be associated with costs, discomforts or impracticalities that influence guideline recommendations. Assigning preferences to treatment outcomes is primarily a matter of opinion and will reflect the values of those involved in this process (Hayward *et al.* 1995). It is therefore important to identify who was involved in assigning values to outcomes. Recommendations may differ depending on the relative emphasis placed on specific benefits, harms and costs

(Hayward *et al.* 1995). Expert panels and consensus groups are often used to determine what a guideline will say. A structured process that includes a balance of research methodologists, practising clinicians and patient representatives increases the likelihood that all important values have been considered (Hayward *et al.* 1995). Variation (disagreement) and uncertainty in values could affect summary recommendations and should be recorded and reported.

Guidelines often concern health care problems about which new knowledge is actively being sought in ongoing studies. It is therefore important to ensure that all current evidence has been considered. As a result of the time required to identify and review a large volume of evidence and achieve consensus about recommendations, guidelines may be out of date by the time they are published. It is helpful if guidelines identify important studies in progress and new information that could change the recommendations made.

People may interpret evidence differently and their values may differ – guidelines are subject to both sorts of differences. Confidence in the validity of a guideline will be increased if external reviewers have judged the conclusions reasonable and other health professionals have found the guidelines applicable in practice. Among guidelines developed by different groups about the same health condition or intervention, there should be little variation in estimates of the strength of evidence as long as the supporting overviews considered the same body of literature. Differences in recommendations probably reflect differences in the relative value placed on various health and economic outcomes in the context of different patient populations and different health care settings.

To be useful, guidelines should give practical, unambiguous advice about specific clinical problems. They should describe the patient population to which recommendations apply, any interventions considered and their optimal role in patient management (Wilson *et al.* 1995). It is important to determine if your patients are the intended target of a particular guideline. To be clinically important, a practice guideline should convince you that the benefits of following the recommendations are worth the expected harms and costs, taking into consideration both the relative and absolute changes in outcomes (Wilson *et al.* 1995). It is also important to consider whether the values assigned to outcomes could differ sufficiently from your patients' preferences to change a decision about whether you adopt a recommendation.

How should clinical practice guidelines be integrated into practice?

No matter how they are developed and implemented, guidelines may do more harm than good if they are inappropriately interpreted or applied. Even excellent external evidence may be inapplicable to, or inappropriate for, an individual patient. A good guideline, based on the best available clinically relevant evidence from systematic research and an explicit process for judging the value of alternative practices, allows you to review the links between different treatment options and outcomes. The integration of this information with individual clinical expertise should determine whether and how it matches the clinical state, predicament and preferences of the individual patient and thus whether it should be applied (Sackett *et al.* 1996).

Implementation of guidelines

Guidelines are not an end in themselves: they are helpful only if they ultimately influence and improve clinical practice. Ensuring appropriate dissemination and implementation of guidelines is critical if they are to change clinical practice. Guidelines will fail to bring about change if they do not reach their intended users. Adequate dissemination is thus necessary for guidelines to be used, but implementation requires active strategies to facilitate changes in behaviour (Thomson *et al.* 1995). A complex set of factors appears to influence the uptake of research findings and a variety of dissemination methods need to be used to encourage health professionals to make informed changes in their practice. Even when findings are summarised and made relevant to the setting in which health professionals will use them, further action is often needed to ensure their implementation. There is some evidence that the greater the educational component of dissemination, the greater is the likelihood that guidelines will be adopted in practice (Grimshaw & Russell 1994). Specific educational interventions based on guidelines and targeted at end users are more likely to be effective than simply posting guidelines or publishing them in professional journals. Promotion and endorsement by peers, particularly respected local clinicians, may also enhance adoption (Thomson *et al.* 1995).

It has been demonstrated repeatedly that the ownership of guidelines by the people who are intended to use them locally is crucial to whether or not guidelines are actually used (Delamothe 1993; Grimshaw & Russell 1993). Local bodies may need to produce their own guidelines even if these are virtually identical to the national models, to ensure ownership and increase the chances of effective dissemination and implementation within particular local contexts. However, guideline development is expensive and local initiatives cannot hope to draw on the same level of scientific resource as those carried out at national level. For this reason, NHS policy in the United Kingdom has promoted the development of national guidelines that can be used as a framework to be modified for local use.

One of the most effective implementation strategies is the use of patient-specific reminders at the time of consultation. These might include attaching guidelines to the medical record, inclusion of guidelines in a computerised patient record or specially designed clinical records. Hayward *et al.* (1995) have suggested that clinicians prefer short manuals or summaries of major recommendations and a synopsis of the underlying evidence that summarises the expected benefits and harms. The key factor is that the guidelines are available at the place and time of clinical decision making and are thus able to influence the clinical decision prospectively (Thomson *et al.* 1995).

It is also important to consider the health care setting in which the guidelines are to be implemented: valid practice guidelines coupled with effective implementation strategies may have no impact if constraints of access, availability or cost are very strong or if attitudinal barriers prevent their endorsement (Tunis *et al.* 1994). A number of factors have been identified that may impede the implementation of guidelines (Lomas & Haynes 1987; Delamothe 1993; Grimshaw & Russell 1993, 1994; Ayers *et al.* 1995; Thomson *et al.* 1995; Newton *et al.* 1996). These include the pressures on health professionals' time, the scale and complexity of some guidelines that need to be adapted on a patient-by- patient basis, lack of co-operation between health professionals required to follow a guideline, making overall control problematic, and difficulty in adjusting guidelines to locally available skills and circumstances because of a lack of investment of local resources. A further barrier may be a lack of consensus among the medical community that guidelines are either necessary or helpful, because of fears that they may compromise clinical freedom.

What evidence is there that guidelines can improve clinical effectiveness?

The application of guidelines should produce improved quality of care for patients associated with measurable improvements in outcomes. However, formal evaluation of the impact of guidelines on practice is rare. Although measurement of improved patient outcomes represents the gold standard of guideline evaluation, this may be impractical. Modification of provider practices and other 'process measures' have been the outcomes most often studied. Although these may be viewed as less important surrogate outcomes, if selected carefully they can be viewed as intermediate steps causally linking recommendations to more meaningful patient-centred outcomes. A systematic review of 59 rigorous studies, evaluating the effect of practice guidelines in the research setting (in which participants were highly selected and evaluation was an explicit part of guideline introduction), found that 55 of them demonstrated significant improvements in the process of care (what doctors did) after the introduction of the guidelines (Grimshaw & Russell 1993). In an update of this review, 12 of 17 studies that measured patient outcome (what happened to patients) after guideline implementation reported a significant improvement in at least one outcome (Grimshaw *et al.* 1995b). However, guidelines do not necessarily improve either performance or outcome. A wide variation in the size of the improvements in performance achieved by clinical guidelines has been demonstrated (Lomas & Haynes 1987; Grimshaw & Russell 1993). Grimshaw and Russell (1993) concluded that the probability of a guideline being effective depended on three factors: the development strategy (where and how guidelines were produced), the dissemination strategy (how they were brought to the attention of clinicians) and the implementation strategy (how the clinician was prompted to follow them). Audit may play a role in evaluating guidelines through a comparison with previous results ('have we improved') or comparison with defined standards (Thomson *et al.* 1995).

Conclusions

Evidence-based clinical practice guidelines, such as those now available for lung cancer (National Health Service Executive 1998; Scottish Intercollegiate Guidelines Network 1998; Royal College of Radiologists' Clinical Oncology Information Network 1999) can assist clinicians in identifying and promoting effective processes of care and treatments. When appropriately disseminated and implemented, they can lead to changes in clinical practice, help to improve the quality of patient care and reduce inappropriate variation in treatment outcomes. As clinical practice guidelines have potential limitations a mechanism is required to formally evaluate their effect on clinical practice and patient outcomes. The ultimate benefit will be to show that health professionals use treatments proved to be of value in clinical trials to the benefit of patients and that all patients achieve the best outcomes reported in the literature.

References

Audet AM, Greenfield S, Field M (1990). Medical practice guidelines: current activities and future directions. *Annals of Internal Medicine* **113**, 709–14

Ayers P, Renvoize T, Robinson M (1995). Clinical Guidelines: key decisions for acute service providers. *British Journal of Health Care Management* **1**, 547–51

Berrino F, Sant M, Verdecchia A, Capocaccia R, Hakulinen T, Esteve J (1995). *Survival of Cancer Patients in Europe. The Eurocare Study.* Geneva: IARC

Cancer Research Campaign (1996). *Lung Cancer and Smoking.* London: CRC

Cluzeau FA, Littlejohns P, Grimshaw JM, Moran SE (1999). Development and application of a generic methodology to assess the quality of clinical guidelines. *International Journal of Quality Health Care* **11**, 21–8

Davis DA, Thomson MA, Oxman AD, Haynes RB (1995). Changing physician performance. A systematic review of the effect of continuing medical education strategies. *Journal of the American Medical Association* **274**, 700–5

Delamothe T (1993). Wanted: guidelines that doctors will follow. *British Medical Journal* **307**, 218

Eddy DM (1990). Clinical decision making. *Journal of the American Medical Association* **264**, 389–91

Freemantle N, Harvey EL, Grimshaw JM *et al.* (1997). The effectiveness of printed educational materials in changing behaviour of health care professionals. *Evidence Based Medicine* **2**, 95

Greengold NL & Weingarten SR (1996). Developing evidence-based practice guidelines and pathways: the experience at the local hospital level. *Jt Comm J Qual Improv* **22**, 391–402

Greenhalgh T (1997). Papers that summarise other papers (systematic reviews and meta-analyses). *Brirtish Medical Journal* **315**, 672–5

Grilli R, Magrini N, Penna A, Mura G, Liberati A (2000). Practice guidelines developed by specialty societies: the need for a critical appraisal. *Lancet* **355**, 103–6

Grimshaw J, Eccles M, Russell I (1995a). Developing clinically valid practice guidelines. *Journal of Evaluation in Clinical Practice* **1**, 37–48

Grimshaw J, Freemantle N, Wallace S *et al.* (1995b). Developing and implementing clinical practice guidelines. *Quality in Health Care* **4**, 55–64

Grimshaw JM & Russell IT (1994). Achieving health gain through guidelines. II. Ensuring guidelines change medical practice. *Quality in Health Care* **3**, 45–52

Grimshaw JM & Russell IT (1993). Effect of clinical guidelines on medical practice: a systematic review of rigorous evaluations. *Lancet* **342**, 1317–22

Haines A & Jones R (1994). Implementing findings of research. *British Medical Journal* **308**, 1488–92

Haward RA (1998). Preparing guidelines and documented clinical policies. *Annals of Oncology* **9**, 1073–8

Haynes RB, Sackett DL, Gray JA *et al.* (1997). Transferring evidence from research into practice: 4. Overcoming barriers to application. *Evidence Based Medicine* **2**, 68w

Hayward RS, Wilson MC, Tunis SR, Bass EB, Guyatt G (1995). Users' guides to the medical literature. VIII. How to use clinical practice guidelines. A. Are the recommendations valid? The Evidence-Based Medicine Working Group. *Journal of the American Medical Association* **274**, 570–4

Jackson R & Feder G (1998). Guidelines for clinical guidelines. A simple, pragmatic strategy for guideline development. *British Medical Journal* **317**, 427–8

Karjalainen S & Palva I (1989). Do treatment protocols improve end results? A study of survival of patients with multiple myeloma in Finland. *British Medical Journal* **299**, 1069–72

Ketley D & Woods KL (1993). Impact of clinical trials on clinical practice: Example of thrombolysis for acute myocardial infarction. *Lancet* **342**, 891–4

Lomas J & Haynes RB (1987). A taxonomy and critical review of tested strategies for the application of clinical practice recommendations. From "official" to "individual" clinical policy. *American Journal of Preventive Medicine* **4**, 77–94

Maher EJ, Timothy A, Squire CJ *et al.* (1993). Audit: The use of radiotherapy for NSCLC in the UK. *Clinical Oncology* **5**, 72–9

Newton J, Knight D, Woolhead G (1996). General practitioners and clinical guidelines: a survey of knowledge, use and beliefs. *British Journal of General Practice* **46**, 513–7

National Health Service Executive (1998). *Guidance on Commissioning Cancer Services. Improving Outcomes in Lung Cancer: the Manual.* Leeds: NHS Executive

Pearson SD, Goulart-Fisher D, Lee TH (1995). Critical pathways as a strategy for improving care: Problems and potential. *Annals of Internal Medicine* **123**, 941–8

Royal College of Radiologists' Clinical Oncology Information Network (1999). Guidelines on the non-surgical management of lung cancer. *Clinical Oncology* **11**, S1–S53

Sackett DL, Rosenberg WMC, Gray JAM, Haynes RM, Richardson WS (1996). Evidence-based medicine: what it is and what it isn't. *British Medical Journal* **312**, 71–2

Scottish Intercollegiate Guidelines Network (1998). *Management of Lung Cancer* (http://pc47.cee.hw.ac.uk/sign/home.htm)

Thomson R, Lavender M, Madhok R (1995). How to ensure that guidelines are effective. *British Medical Journal* **311**, 237–42

Tunis SR, Hayward RS, Wilson MC *et al.* (1994). Internists' attitudes about clinical practice guidelines. *Annals of Internal Medicine* **120**, 956–63

West E & Newton J (1997). Clinical guidelines. An ambitious national strategy. *British Medical Journal* **315**, 324

Wilson MC, Hayward RS, Tunis SR, Bass EB, Guyatt G (1995). Users' guides to the Medical Literature. VIII. How to use clinical practice guidelines. B. What are the recommendations and will they help you in caring for your patients? The Evidence-Based Medicine Working Group. *Journal of the American Medical Association* **274**, 1630–2

Winstanley JH, Leinster SJ, Wake PN, Copeland GP (1995). The value of guidelines in a breast screening service. *European Journal of Surgical Oncology* **21,** 140–2

Delivering effective services efficiently: current models of excellence for the provision of an efficient service

Clare Laroche and Erica Lowry

Introduction

Cancer registry data suggest that five-year survival rates for many cancers are significantly lower in the UK than in other European countries (Sikora 1999). Lung cancer is the most frequently occurring cancer in the UK, accounting for 21 per cent of all male cancers and 12 per cent of all female cancers. In 1994, lung cancer represented 15 per cent of all new cancers and 23 per cent of all cancer deaths, with a five-year survival rate significantly lower than that reported for the rest of Europe and the USA. In the UK, five-year survival appears to be around 5 per cent (NHS Centre for Reviews and Dissemination 1998), as compared to an overall five-year survival in the USA of around 13 per cent (Fry *et al.* 1999). The cause for this discrepancy is not clear-cut. However, analysis of the USA Cancer Registry reports show clearly how survival is linked to surgical resection (Fry *et al.*1999).

It has long been recognised that, in the UK, services for patients with lung cancer have been disorganised and under-resourced, with low rates of histological diagnosis (Melling *et al.* 1998), especially in the elderly (Brown *et al.* 1996), striking variations in management even between specialists (Fergusson *et al.* 1996) and fewer than expected patients being referred for radical treatments, particularly potentially curative surgery (Standing Medical Advisory Committee 1994; Damhuis & Schutte 1996; Moghissi & Connolly 1996; Muers & Haward 1996; Pickles & Rudolf 1996) Over the past five years, considerable effort has been made to establish a more uniform investigation and treatment pathway for patients with lung cancer in the UK (George 1997).

Specialist nursing expertise is integral to the effective management of patients via any rapid access lung cancer service, as outlined in the 1998 Department of Health guidelines (NHS Executive 1998a). The need for strong clinical leadership from cancer nurses has been further endorsed by a recent NHS Executive document (NHS Executive 2000). The specialist nurse requires sound knowledge of the cancer process, the treatment options available and the spectrum of services which can be accessed. The nurse must possess the skills necessary to support patients facing a life-threatening illness.

Presentation of lung cancer

Lung cancer currently still has a low profile within the general population, despite the recent efforts of some celebrities with the disease. More education of the general public is needed to ensure that people in high risk groups are aware of the need to seek advice promptly if they experience suggestive symptoms, especially haemoptysis. Similarly, discussion and training is required in primary care to ensure that such patients are dealt with appropriately.

It is recognised that patients often delay seeking medical advice about symptoms suggestive of lung cancer. A study from Nottingham showed that there could be a delay of several weeks between the onset of symptoms and a patient seeing their GP (Scriven *et al.*1999). This was true even for patients with haemoptysis. It is not clear whether this is due to a lack of knowledge within the general population, or to patient denial resulting from the general public perception of the poor prognosis for lung cancer. However, in addition to the attempts currently being made to speed up the investigation of patients after presentation, these other delays need to be considered.

The main symptoms of lung cancer, in particular haemoptysis, increased shortness of breath, chest pains, cough, weight loss and lack of energy are all common symptoms in primary care, and are by no means specific. The recent inclusion of lung cancer patients in the 'two week wait' government initiative has meant that guidelines will need to be developed locally both to ensure that patients at highest risk are investigated promptly, and that patients at low risk do not clog up an often overloaded system. Without clear guidelines it may be difficult for a GP to decide which patients to refer to secondary care for urgent investigation. Preliminary advice recommends that GPs should perform an urgent chest radiograph (CXR) in all patients with suspicious symptoms. They should then refer urgently (within the two week deadline) those with an abnormal CXR or those with obvious symptoms of proximal large airways obstruction i.e., stridor or significant on-going haemoptysis. However it is important for GPs to be aware that as many as 5 per cent of patients with lung cancer present with a normal CXR, and that such patients often experience significant delay in accessing secondary care. It will therefore be necessary for patients with ongoing suspicious symptoms to be referred for a chest clinic appointment even if the initial chest radiograph appears normal.

Current models of service could therefore potentially be made more effective by educating people at high risk of lung cancer to recognise suspicious symptoms in primary care, and providing GPs with a clear route to access appropriate screening investigations.

Delivering an effective service

An effective service for lung cancer patients should rapidly identify all patients suitable for potentially curative treatment, identify palliative and social care needs early in the patient journey (and then deliver them), and provide all necessary active treatments within agreed acceptable timescales (NHS Centre for Reviews and Dissemination 1998). However, previous studies suggest that this type of service has not been available for many patients with suspected lung cancer in the UK (Fergusson *et al.* 1999). In 1996, Billing & Wells published figures from the Papworth Surgical Unit to suggest that the mean total delay between presentation and potentially curative surgery was 109 days. Within this period, an average of one month occurred before referral to a respiratory specialist who then spent two months investigating the patient.

Within the last few years, many UK centres have redesigned their lung cancer services in an attempt to improve efficiency although published evidence of improved outcomes remains scanty. In 1998, the Department of Health published guidelines on the organisation of care for patients with lung cancer (NHS Executive 1998a), although they recognised that many of the recommendations were not fully supported by scientific evidence.

In 1995, Papworth and Addenbrookes hospitals in Cambridge set up a new combined thoracic oncology unit, providing a comprehensive lung cancer service to the three surrounding health districts. Three new sessions of respiratory physician time were obtained; a new thoracic surgeon was appointed at the cardiothoracic unit at Papworth, and a new oncologist was appointed across the two sites specialising in lung cancer. Patients were referred to the service by any of the local respiratory physicians after initial assessment in the patient's local district hospital. Notes and radiographs were reviewed jointly at Papworth by the respiratory physician co-ordinating the service, and by a specialist respiratory radiologist. Patients were provisionally assigned to either a bronchoscopy or percutaneous needle biopsy on the next investigation day, and were informed of their investigation day timetable by a phone call from one of the day unit nurses. On arrival in the Papworth thoracic day unit, they underwent a computed tomographic (CT) assessment of thorax and upper abdomen as the initial investigation. On the basis of this they either proceeded to the planned investigation, or, since the two lists were running simultaneously, they could be switched to the alternative invasive investigation if this was thought more likely to give a tissue diagnosis on the basis of the CT scan. Other investigations required for staging or assessment of fitness for radical treatment were also performed at this stage, on the basis of symptoms and/or previous medical history (e.g., for staging: bone scan, CT scan of head etc; for fitness: ECG, full lung function, echocardiogram, cardiac exercise test etc).

In the Papworth and Addenbrookes' service, specialist nursing input commenced in January 1996 via a hospital-based post funded initially by Macmillan Cancer Relief. The nurse follows the patient through their cancer journey facilitating understanding and acting as a point of reference at times of uncertainty. The aim is to personalise the service and enable patients to retain a sense of control. Specialist nurses now move between the two hospitals to facilitate continuity of care. During the initial investigation day the nurse makes a preliminary assessment of key needs and reviews symptom control. Involvement prior to diagnosis enables anticipatory planning of care and is a crucial feature of the service.

In the Papworth and Addenbrookes' service, all patients are discussed in a multidisciplinary meeting held three days after the investigation day, and a provisional management plan is formulated. Further investigations can also be organised at this point so that most necessary information is available when the patient is first seen in the follow-up clinic. The benefit of performing all investigations in a co-ordinated way in the cardiothoracic centre allows ready access to all necessary investigations with the minimum of delay. Patients are seen in a combined clinic the following week to receive their diagnosis and discuss the management plan. This strategy ensures that all patients are reviewed by both an oncologist and a thoracic surgeon and that delays between presentation and diagnosis, and between diagnosis and an appointment with the appropriate specialist for treatment, are minimised.

It is recognised that the way in which patients hear their diagnosis impacts significantly on the rest of their cancer journey (Buckman 1992). At Papworth patients are seen in a nursing consultation which follows the medical discussion of diagnosis and management. Information giving is secondary to the empathetic support offered. The majority of patients are referred to district nurses and some to community Macmillan teams. Other hospital and community professionals may also be involved. A telephone helpline is available to patients, family members and colleagues.

Results from the first 275 patients investigated in the Papworth and Addenbrookes' service showed that, of the 181 patients with confirmed non-small cell lung cancer, 25 per cent underwent successful surgical resection, with a failed thoracotomy rate of 11 per cent, and a median time from initial chest clinic appointment to surgery of five weeks (Laroche *et al.* 1998). The new service was associated with a significant increase in the absolute number of patients undergoing surgical resection for lung cancer at Papworth. However, since an unknown proportion of patients with lung cancer in the three health districts was being investigated outside the service, the overall proportion of patients undergoing resection is uncertain. Further analysis, looking at cancer registry and hospital coding data will be necessary in order to assess how many patients are being managed outside of the service, and whether the new service has a significant impact on outcomes in the total lung cancer population in each health district. A new Management of Breathlessness Clinic was established in 1999. Experienced cancer and palliative care nurses play a vital role in promoting a coherent and sensitive service for this group of patients.

A similar service in Liverpool, incorporating a rapid access clinic and dedicated CT sessions, was associated with an increase in surgical resection rate from 12 per cent to 21 per cent, suggesting that it may be universal CT scanning which has the most impact on surgical resection rate (Warburton *et al.* 1999).

Efficiency of invasive lung cancer investigations

Until recently, most patients referred with symptoms suggesting an endobronchial carcinoma would undergo a bronchoscopy as their first investigation after a clinical assessment and chest radiograph. However, in approximately 25 per cent of patients subsequently confirmed as having lung cancer, initial bronchoscopy will be non-diagnostic (Royal College of Physicians 1999). Papworth have recently reported the results of a randomised two group study to assess the effectiveness of performing an initial CT scan in patients with suspected lung cancer (Laroche *et al.* 2000). One hundred and seventy one patients with suspected endobronchial carcinoma, provisionally booked for a bronchoscopy, underwent an initial staging CT scan of thorax and upper abdomen. Patients with an obvious peripheral lesion on their chest radiograph, suitable for percutaneous biopsy, were excluded. One group of patients (group B) underwent bronchoscopy as planned, with the bronchoscopist blinded to the result of the CT scan until immediately after the procedure, whereas the other group of patients (group A) underwent whichever investigation was thought most likely to give a tissue diagnosis on the basis of the CT scan. The study showed that, in patients with confirmed lung cancer, an initial CT scan increased the chance of obtaining a tissue diagnosis on initial invasive investigation from 71 per cent to 90 per cent ($p=0.004$), and increased the chance of obtaining a positive result from bronchoscopy from 71 per cent to 89 per cent ($p=0.012$).

Economic evaluation also showed that this strategy was cost neutral, if one asumed that around 60 per cent of patients would normally have a staging CT scan at some stage in the investigation process anyway. However, in areas of the country where CT scanning is not performed routinely in most patients (Fergusson *et al.* 1996), there would obviously be a cost implication in this approach.

The provision of early, universal CT staging before bronchoscopy will require some reorganisation of services. One model would entail performing a staging CT scan on the day of initial chest clinic appointment, allowing selection of the most appropriate initial invasive investigation to be performed on the next investigation day. This would minimise wasted bronchoscopy slots, but perhaps could result in an increased rate of unnecessary CT scans. Some centres have already established a direct access approach, with patients undergoing bronchoscopy on the same day (Deegan *et al.* 1998; Williams *et al.* 1999). This has the advantage of minimising the time between first consultation and investigation and also, potentially, the number of hospital visits, although in one centre, the reservation of same-day slots for patients assessed as potentially needing bronchoscopy from the referral letter resulted in up to half such slots being wasted. One relatively small centre combined same day CT scans and bronchoscopy on the day of initial chest clinic review (Williams *et al.* 1999).

The importance of the multidisciplinary team

Both the Calman-Hine report on Cancer Services (1995), and subsequent documents focusing specifically on lung cancer (NHS Executive 1998a; Scottish Intercollegiate Guidelines Network 1998; The Lung Cancer Working Party of the British Thoracic Society 1998; Clinical Oncology Information Network 1999), have emphasised the importance of the multidisciplinary team. However evidence for their effectiveness is scanty in lung cancer. Potential benefits would be the increased surgical and oncological input into every patient, and also the easier application of applying multidisciplinary treatments. However in units investigating fewer than 300 patients a year, without an on-site cardiothoracic surgical service, the provision of surgical input into every lung cancer patient may be difficult to justify on an economic basis.

In Southend this problem has been overcome with the use of a telemedicine clinic, using the transmission of radiographic images from the multidisciplinary clinic in the district general hospital to a specialist centre for review by cardiothoracic surgeon and thoracic radiologist (Davison et al. 1999).

Entry into clinical trials

Very few patients with lung cancer are entered into any form of clinical trial. This is true both in Europe and the US (Krasna et al. 1999). There are many reasons for this, including the poor prognosis of most patients, their poor performance status at presentation, the lack of suitable trials for many patients who are already in the palliative stages of their disease at presentation, and a lack of time and personnel in busy lung cancer clinics. One of the benefits of a larger service managing a significant number of lung cancer patients per year, is that it is easier to justify the appointment of additional personnel to co-ordinate and manage clinical trials. Evidence from Papworth suggests that this approach may ultimately increase the overall proportion of patients entering a clinical trial (Magee et al. 1999).

Conclusions

Reasons for the poor survival figures for lung cancer patients in the UK compared to Europe and the USA are not certain. However it is clear that in many regions of the UK, access to appropriate investigations, treatment and palliative care is unsatisfactory. Active assessment of local resources and health needs is required throughout the UK to ensure that patients presenting with suspicious symptoms can receive an equal level of care throughout the country. In some areas this may require a considerable reorganisation of services and increase in resources, although, as several centres have shown recently, such reorganisation can result in significant improvements in the standard of patient investigation which may, in the longterm, be associated with improvements in outcome.

References

Billing JS & Wells FC (1996). Delays in the diagnosis and surgical treatment of lung cancer. *Thorax* **51,** 903–6

Brown JS, Eraut D, Trask C, Davidson A (1996). Age and the treatment of lung cancer. *Thorax* **51,** 564–8

Buckman R (1992). *How to Break Bad News.* London: Pan Books

Clinical Oncology Information Network (1999). *Guidelines on the Non-Surgical Management of Lung Cancer.* London: Royal College of Radiologists

Damhuis RAM & Schütte PR (1996). Resection rates and postoperative mortality in 7,899 patients with lung cancer. *European Respiratory Journal* **9,** 7–10

Davison AG, Eraut CD, Khan N *et al.* (1999). Telemedicine for lung cancer: A new multidisciplinary approach. *Thorax* **54,** A 37

Deegan PC, Heath L, Brunskill J, Kinnear WJM, Morgan SA , Johnston IDA (1998). Reducing waiting times in lung cancer. *Journal of the Royal College of Physician of London* **32,** 339–43

Fergusson RJ, Gregor A, Dodds R, Kerr G (1996). Management of lung cancer on South East Scotland. *Thorax* **51,** 569–74

Fergusson RJ, Milroy R, Brown P, Gregor A, Jones R, Stroner PL (1999). Lung cancer in Scotland – importance of seeing a Chest Physician. *Thorax* **54,** A34

Fry WA, Phillips JL, Menck HR (1999). Ten-year survey of lung cancer treatment and survival in hospitals in the United States. *Cancer* **86,** 1867–76

George PJM (1997). Delays in the management of lung cancer *Thorax* **52,** 107–8

Krasna MJ, Reed CE, Nugent WC *et al.* (1999). Lung cancer staging and treatment in multidisciplinary trials: cancer and leukemia Group B co-operative group approach. *Annals of Thoracic Surgery* **68,** 201–7

Krishnasamy M & Wilkie E (1997). Lung cancer: patients', families' amd professionals' perceptions of health care need. A national needs assessment study. Macmillan Cancer Relief Nov (unpublished)

Laroche C, Fairburn I, Moss H *et al.* (2000). Role of computed tomographic scanning of the thorax prior to bronchoscopy in the investigation of suspected lung cancer. *Thorax* **55,** 359–63

Laroche C, Wells F, Coulden R *et al.* (1998). Improving surgical resection rate in lung cancer. *Thorax* **53,** 445–9

Magee L, Laroche C, Gilligan D (1999). Clinical trials in lung cancer: Can a programmed investigation unit and a multidisciplinary clinic help? *Thorax* **54,** A35

Melling PP, Round CE, Muers MF *et al.* (1998). Lung cancer referral patterns. *Thorax* **53,** A 25

Moghissi K & Connolly C K (1996). Resection rates in lung cancer patients. *European Respiratory Journal* **9,** 5–6

Muers MF & Haward RA (1996). Management of lung cancer. *Thorax* **51,** 557–60

NHS Centre for Reviews and Dissemination, University of York (1998). Management of lung cancer. *Effective Health Care* **4,** 1–12

NHS Executive (1998a). *Guidance on Commissioning Cancer Services: Improving Outcomes in Lung Cancer – the Manual.* Leeds: Department of Health

NHS Executive (1998b). *Guidance on Commissioning Cancer Services: Improving Outcomes in Lung Cancer – the Research Evidence.* Leeds: Department of Health

NHS Executive (2000). *The Nursing Contribution to Cancer Care.* London: Department of Health

Pickles H & Rudolf M (1996). Lung cancer: local review of services. *Thorax* **5,** A 57

Royal College of Physicians Clinical Effectiveness and Evaluation Unit (1999). *Lung Cancer Audit*. London: Royal College of Physicians

Scottish Intercollegiate Guidelines Network (1998). *Management of Lung Cancer.* SIGN publication no 23. Edinburgh: Royal College of Physicians

Scriven NA, Johnston I, Kinnear W (1999). How long do patients have symptoms before presenting to hospital? *Thorax* **54,** A35

Sikora K (1999). Cancer survival in Britain. *British Medical Journal* **319,** 461–2

Standing Medical Advisory Committee (1994). *Management of Lung Cancer: Current Clinical Practices.* London: Department of Health

The Lung Cancer Working Party of the British Thoracic Society (1998). British Thoracic Society recommendations to respiratory physicians for organising the care of patients with lung cancer. *Thorax* **53,** S1–8

Warburton CJ, Ryland I, Earis JE (1999). Improved surgical resection rate as a result of changes in organisation of lung cancer services. *Thorax* **54,** A37

Williams TJ, Clearkin RJ, Walter DF, Lavelle LA , Birring SS (1999). A one-stop CT/Bronchoscopy clinic for patients with suspected lung cancer: A District General Hospital experience. *Thorax* **54,** A34

Index